THE DIET APPROACH FOR BEATING CUSHING'S DISEASE

A Comprehensive Guide for Gaining Control of Your Weight, Reversing Symptoms of Hypercortisolism, and Other Pituitary Diseases

Zara Anderson M.D.

COPYRIGHT PAGE

PLEASE READ

Table of Contents

CHAPTER 1: UNDERSTANDING CUSHING'S DISEASE

Hypercortisolism, commonly known as Cushing's disease, is a very unusual endocrine ailment in which the body produces too much of the stress hormone cortisol. Pituitary adenomas, benign tumours of the gland at the brain's base, are to blame. Adrenocorticotropic hormone (ACTH) is overproduced by this tumour, leading to excessive cortisol production.

The hormone cortisol is essential for maintaining proper metabolic, immunological, and stress

1

responses, among other things. However, in Cushing's disease, elevated cortisol levels cause havoc with bodily processes and contribute to a wide variety of signs and symptoms.

Weight increase (especially in the face, neck, and belly), wasting (especially in the arms and legs), and acne are the most typical manifestations of Cushing's illness. Patients may gain weight in the abdomen and torso, resulting in a "buffalo hump" and a "moon face." Stretch marks, acne, and easily bruised skin are among other possible physical signs.

Cushing's illness also causes widespread changes in metabolism and hormone levels. Some of the risk factors for bone fractures are: hypertension, diabetes, muscular weakness, and osteoporosis. Mood swings, anger, anxiety, and sadness are all possible side effects of high cortisol in patients.

Cushing's disease is diagnosed after a thorough review that includes a patient's medical history, a physical examination, and other diagnostic procedures. Imaging examinations, such as MRI or CT scans, assist localise the pituitary tumour, while blood and urine tests evaluate cortisol and ACTH levels. The diagnosis may be confirmed with further testing, such as the dexamethasone suppression test.

Cushing's disease treatment choices are condition-and severity-specific. Pituitary tumours are often treated with transsphenoidal surgery, which entails removing the tumour through the nasal passages. Medication to inhibit cortisol production or radiation therapy may be alternatives to surgery if the former is not an option.

Cushing's illness is best treated by a team of specialists, including endocrinologists, neurosurgeons, and others. The goals of treatment are symptom relief, restoration of normal cortisol levels, and prevention of consequences. Long-term illness care requires constant attention, including monthly check-ins, hormone monitoring, and dietary and physical activity adjustments.

Early identification and treatment of Cushing's disease can help reduce symptoms and boost overall quality of life, despite the condition's severe impact on a person's physical and mental well-being. Anyone having symptoms they find troubling should make an appointment with a doctor for assessment and advice.

Prevalence of Cushing's Disease

Cushing's disease is uncommon, affecting just around 10 to 15 persons out of every million. Women make up around 70% to 80% of those diagnosed with this condition, although men are not immune. Although it may affect anyone of any age, those between the ages of 20 and 50 tend to be the focus of diagnoses.

Although Cushing's illness is thought to be uncommon, its true frequency may be underreported due to diagnostic difficulties. Cushing's illness is notoriously tricky to diagnose due to the subtlety of its symptoms and the fact that they often coincide with those of other disorders. There may be gaps in diagnosis and underreporting of instances because of the various tests and examinations that are often part of the diagnostic procedure.

There may be a greater incidence of Cushing's illness in some communities. Cushing's disease is more likely to occur in people who have certain risk factors, such as a family history of pituitary adenomas or a genetic abnormality like multiple endocrine neoplasia type 1 (MEN1).

Although Cushing's disease is somewhat common, Cushing's syndrome, which includes Cushing's disease and other causes of hypercortisolism, is more common. This is due to the fact that adrenal tumours and ectopic ACTH-producing tumours are also potential causes of Cushing's syndrome, in addition to pituitary adenomas.

Although Cushing's illness is very uncommon, it is critical that it be better recognised and diagnosed so that patients can be diagnosed and treated as soon as possible.

Causes and Risk Factors

Cushing's disease is caused by a benign tumour in the pituitary gland called an adenoma. The adrenal glands generate an abundance of cortisol because of the tumor's effect on adrenocorticotropic hormone (ACTH). However, it has yet to be determined what causes pituitary adenomas to form.

Cushing's disease has been linked to a few specific causes. The illness strikes between the ages of 30 and 50 with greater frequency among women than males. Family history of pituitary tumours or genetic abnormalities like multiple endocrine neoplasia type 1 (MEN1) or Carney complex may further enhance the risk.

Cushing's illness may potentially arise from ectopic ACTH production in some people. Excess cortisol is produced when tumours in locations other than the pituitary gland (such the lungs or pancreas) secrete ACTH. Small cell lung cancer and carcinoid tumours are frequently linked to these growths.

In addition to Cushing's disease, Cushing's syndrome can develop through long-term usage of glucocorticoid drugs like prednisone or dexamethasone. Differentiating between exogenous (drug-induced) and endogenous (tumor-induced) causes of increased cortisol production is crucial for accurate diagnosis and treatment.

Overproduction of ACTH and cortisol due to the existence of a pituitary adenoma is the primary cause of Cushing's disease, while the precise causes remain unknown. In order to effectively treat Cushing's illness, it is essential to first pinpoint its underlying causes.

Signs and Symptoms

There is a significant variety in the intensity of symptoms experienced by people with Cushing's illness. High cortisol levels in the body cause these symptoms by damaging many organs.

The upper torso, face, and neck tend to acquire weight first, whereas the limbs may stay relatively slender. This causes a rise in abdominal fat and a round or "moon-shaped" face, as well as a fatty "buffalo hump" between the shoulders. Muscle weakness and skin fragility, making bruises easier to appear, are further symptoms of Cushing's illness.

Excessive cortisol production can induce a hormonal imbalance, which in turn can cause a number of undesirable effects. One such condition is hypertension, which raises the danger of cardiovascular diseases including heart attack and stroke. Alterations in menstrual cycles and libido are two additional symptoms of hormonal imbalance.

Elevated blood sugar levels and an increased chance of developing diabetes are both side effects of Cushing's illness, which can also impair the body's metabolism. Depression, irritability, and mood swings are other symptoms. An reduced ability to heal wounds or an increased susceptibility to infections have been reported.

Bone health can be negatively impacted by Cushing's disease, leading to osteoporosis and an increased risk of fractures. Stretch marks are another potential side effect, especially on the breasts, buttocks, and tummy. These stretch marks, which might be purple or pink, can be upsetting to those who have them.

Cushing's disease symptoms may be vague and appear gradually over time; this makes it easy for them to be misdiagnosed. Therefore, endocrinologists and specialists in hormone-related illnesses, among others, are required for accurate diagnosis and management of the condition. In order to alleviate symptoms and prevent long-term problems, early diagnosis and treatment is essential.

CHAPTER 2: DIAGNOSIS AND TREATMENT APPROACHES

Cushing's disease can be diagnosed after a thorough assessment including a clinical exam, laboratory testing, and imaging. A proper diagnosis is essential for effective treatment because of the condition's intricacy and the overlap of symptoms with those of other conditions.

Diagnosing Cushing's disease begins with a comprehensive patient history and physical exam. The doctor will examine the patient's medical history, take note of the patient's current

16

symptoms, and ask about the use of any supplements or other treatments the patient may be receiving. After this, cortisol levels in the body will be assessed in a lab.

The overnight dexamethasone suppression test (DST) is the gold standard for diagnosing Cushing's illness. The patient gets a small dosage of the synthetic steroid dexamethasone before bed, and the following morning their cortisol levels are tested. Cortisol levels are not kept in check normally in people with Cushing's disease.

Further diagnostic procedures are carried out to pinpoint the cause of cortisol overproduction if the

DST indicates the existence of excessive cortisol production. Cortisol and other hormone levels, including adrenocorticotropic hormone (ACTH), which is often increased in Cushing's illness, may be measured using blood and urine testing.

The origin of elevated cortisol levels may also be determined by imaging techniques. Magnetic resonance imaging (MRI) is the gold standard for visualising the pituitary gland. This allows for the detection of any pituitary tumours or anomalies that may be responsible for the overproduction of ACTH.

Computed tomography (CT) scans and adrenal vein sample are two further imaging techniques that may be necessary to properly diagnose Cushing's syndrome and rule out other potential causes.

Note that endocrinologists and other experts may be needed for help with the diagnosing procedure for Cushing's illness. Accurate diagnosis and management of the ailment need close coordination between healthcare specialists and a thorough examination.

Treatment Options

Normalising cortisol levels and relieving the symptoms caused by excessive cortisol production are the goals of treatment for Cushing's disease. Treatment strategies might shift based on what's causing the condition, how severe the symptoms are, and other factors unique to each patient.

Cushing's illness often requires surgical intervention. When pituitary tumours are to blame for excessive ACTH production, the most frequent surgical approach is transsphenoidal surgery to remove the tumours. This minimally invasive technique eliminates the necessity for an external incision by gaining access to the pituitary gland through the nose tube. If adrenal tumours are to blame for the body's excessive production of cortisol, then extra surgery may be necessary.

Medical treatment may be undertaken if surgical surgery is either not an option or is ineffective. The effects of cortisol can be reduced or eliminated altogether with the help of certain medications. Ketoconazole and metyrapone are two examples of adrenal enzyme inhibitors that can lower cortisol levels. Cabergoline and pasireotide are two drugs that can be used to either limit the adrenal glands' reaction to ACTH or prevent ACTH from being produced.

When conventional methods, such as surgery and medication, have failed to bring down elevated cortisol levels, radiation therapy may be the next best option. Pituitary or adrenal tumours can be treated with this method by receiving targeted radiation.

Depending on the severity of Cushing's illness, it may be essential to use a combination of therapies. Surgery followed by medication or radiation therapy is one example of a multimodal treatment plan.

Modifying one's way of life can be a powerful tool in the fight against Cushing's illness. This includes things like not smoking, going to the doctor regularly, and taking any medications as directed. The success of therapy, the optimal dosage of any prescribed drugs, and the presence or absence of any adverse effects can only be determined by regular follow-up visits with a healthcare professional.

Patients with Cushing's disease must collaborate closely with their healthcare providers, such as endocrinologists, neurosurgeons, radiologists, and others, to get the best possible treatment outcomes and long-term management of the disease.

Management Strategies and Lifestyle Changes

Cushing's illness requires a multifaceted approach to therapy, including management tactics and lifestyle adjustments for effective long-term control. Maintaining regular medication intake is crucial for successful cortisol management. Relaxation exercises and other stress-reducing activities can also be helpful in reducing the severity of symptoms.

Cushing's disease management is greatly aided by eating well. A healthy diet should consist of a wide range of plant-based foods, as well as whole grains, lean meats, and water. These foods are high in nutrients and can help with weight control, general health, and vitamin and mineral intake.

People with Cushing's disease can benefit greatly from engaging in regular exercise, provided they do so under medical supervision. Helps maintain a healthy weight, boosts exercise, and benefits the heart. When deciding how much and what kind of exercise to do, it's best to talk to a doctor about your specific needs and limitations.

Avoiding tobacco products and cutting down on alcohol use are other important health measures to take. Cigarette smoke is harmful to the body and can make Cushing's disease symptoms worse.

However, alcohol use can compromise the effectiveness of medications and has been linked to weight gain and other health problems.

Appointments with healthcare providers should be scheduled at regular intervals to assess the patient's response to therapy and make any required modifications. The stress hormone cortisol must be tracked, medicines must be evaluated, and any emerging symptoms must be addressed.

Patients with Cushing's disease can improve their health and quality of life by adopting these treatment measures and making some adjustments to their daily habits. Better health outcomes and enhanced quality of life can be achieved via strong collaboration with healthcare practitioners and a proactive attitude to self-care.

Potential Complications

Complications from Cushing's disease are potentially serious and must be closely monitored and managed. Osteoporosis, cardiovascular problems, diabetes, infections, and psychological and emotional effects are only some of the prevalent repercussions of this disorder.

Bone loss and an increased risk of osteoporosis can occur after prolonged exposure to high cortisol. It may be required to monitor bone density on a regular basis and take appropriate action, such as increasing calcium and vitamin D consumption, engaging in weight-bearing workouts, and maybe even taking medication.

Hypertension (high blood pressure), dyslipidemia (abnormal blood lipid levels), and an elevated risk of cardiovascular disease may all be associated with Cushing's illness. Modifications to one's way of life, including eating well, getting plenty of exercise, and controlling risk factors like smoking and weight gain, can have a significant effect on the cardiovascular system.

Increased susceptibility to diabetes has been linked to impaired glucose metabolism caused by chronically elevated cortisol levels. It is crucial to keep track of blood sugar levels and work closely with medical professionals to control them through diet, exercise, and, if necessary, medication.

Due to a compromised immune system, people with Cushing's disease may be at a higher risk of contracting infections. Keeping up with regular cleaning and immunisations, as well as quickly diagnosing and treating any diseases that may arise, are all crucial.

The emotional and mental toll of dealing with Cushing's illness is not to be underestimated. Seeking help from healthcare experts and mental health services is crucial for addressing emotional difficulties and learning coping mechanisms.

The negative effects of these difficulties on one's health can be mitigated by preventative measures and routine medical checkups. In order to properly manage the difficulties of Cushing's disease and improve quality of life, constant collaboration with a multidisciplinary healthcare team is essential.

CHAPTER 3: CUSHING'S DISEASE AND DIET

Overproduction of the hormone cortisol is a hallmark of Cushing's disease, a complicated endocrine illness. Dietary changes, in addition to conventional medical treatment, are essential in the management of Cushing's disease symptoms and the improvement of general health. A healthy and nutritious diet can aid in controlling cortisol levels, maintaining a healthy weight, managing co-morbidities, and improving general health.

Maintaining a healthy ratio of macronutrients is essential for patients with Cushing's disease.

Blood sugar levels and weight control can be supported by a diet that places an emphasis on whole grains, lean protein sources, and healthy fats while minimising processed carbs and saturated fats. Supporting different biological processes and mitigating shortages that may emerge due to the disease or its treatment requires an adequate intake of vital micronutrients, such as vitamins and minerals.

Individuals with Cushing's illness would do well to increase their fibre consumption because of the positive effects it has on digestion, blood sugar regulation, and feeling full. Getting enough fibre in your diet is as simple as eating a wide range of fruits, vegetables, whole grains, and legumes.

Managing symptoms like excessive thirst, enhancing kidney health, and supporting general body functioning all depend on getting enough fluids and staying hydrated.

Foods high in antioxidants and phytonutrients, such as those found in a broad variety of fruits and vegetables, as well as whole grains like quinoa and brown rice, are highly recommended. Milk and other dairy products, or calcium-fortified equivalents, can help people get the calcium they need.

On the other hand, people with Cushing's disease should limit or avoid eating a few specific foods. As they can all contribute to fluid retention, weight gain, and other metabolic issues related to the condition, high-sodium diets, processed and fast foods, sugary beverages, overly fatty foods, and alcohol should be avoided or consumed in moderation.

Managing Cushing's disease requires a systematic approach, including meal planning and quantity management. Stabilising blood sugar levels and managing weight can be accomplished by the preparation of well-balanced meals that include a variety of macronutrients, the careful monitoring of portion sizes, and the maintenance of regular and regulated eating patterns. Preparing meals ahead of time can be helpful, as can cooking techniques that cut back on sugar and fat.

It is highly encouraged to work with a trained dietitian to create a personalised eating plan, track progress, and make any required modifications. The success of the dietary approach in controlling Cushing's disease can be increased via frequent follow-up with healthcare practitioners, the incorporation of lifestyle adjustments including regular physical exercise and stress management strategies, and the pursuit of support from communities that are accepting of those with the condition.

Due to the fact that each patient's illness and treatment plan is unique, it is essential that patients always consult with their doctors before making any significant dietary changes. They may tailor their advice to your specific needs and make sure that any dietary adjustments you make complement your larger Cushing's disease treatment plan.

Role of Diet in Managing Cushing's Disease

Diet plays a significant part in the treatment of Cushing's illness, which is characterised by the body's inordinate production of cortisol. A change in diet will not cure a condition, but it can help manage symptoms, improve health, and boost the efficacy of other treatments. Cortisol levels, body weight, the risk of problems, and overall health outcomes can all benefit from a well-planned and balanced diet.

Keeping blood sugar levels steady is a primary goal of the diet for Cushing's disease patients. This is achieved by eating foods high in complex carbs, such whole grains, legumes, and vegetables, which release glucose slowly into the bloodstream. Lean proteins, such as those found in poultry, fish, and plant foods, can aid in muscle repair and maintenance.

Weight control is a key component of the diet for Cushing's disease. An unhealthy diet might hinder your efforts to maintain your weight, which is a typical indication of the illness. Maintaining a healthy weight may be aided by placing an emphasis on portion management, eating meals high in nutrients, and cutting out on high-calorie and processed options.

Antioxidant- and anti-inflammatory-rich foods should also be included. Fruits and vegetables, especially those with deep hues, are packed with these healthful chemicals. They provide a broad variety of vitamins and minerals and can aid in inflammation reduction and immune system support.

Dietary changes may be recommended by medical practitioners to treat symptoms of Cushing's disease and its possible consequences. If you have hypertension, your doctor may recommend cutting back on salt in your diet. Similarly, those with osteoporosis may benefit from an upped calcium and vitamin D consumption.

Individuals with Cushing's disease should consult with their healthcare team, including trained dietitians, to create a nutrition plan that is personalised to their unique requirements and goals. They may tailor their advice to each individual's needs, keep tabs on how things are going, and make any required alterations to the dietary plan.

Although food is crucial, it should be part of a larger management strategy that also involves seeing a doctor regularly, taking any necessary medications, engaging in regular physical exercise, reducing stress, and getting enough sleep. One can achieve the best possible health results and enhance their quality of life by taking a comprehensive approach to controlling Cushing's disease.

Nutritional Considerations for Cushing's Disease

Management of Cushing's disease, a disorder marked by elevated cortisol levels, is greatly aided by eating well. While dietary changes alone cannot reverse disease progression, they can reduce symptoms, boost health in general, and even make certain medications more effective.

Fluid retention and hypertension can be managed in part by limiting salt consumption. The key is to focus on eating whole, fresh foods that are naturally low in salt rather than relying on processed and packaged options. You may also limit your sodium intake by seasoning your food with herbs and spices rather than salt.

Since Cushing's illness can lead to potassium depletion, it's crucial to include potassium-rich items in the diet. Bananas, oranges, dark green vegetables, and avocados are all high-potassium foods. The potassium in these meals can help keep your heart healthy and pumping strong.

Because of the increased risk of bone loss and osteoporosis, it is essential for people with Cushing's disease to maintain a sufficient diet of calcium and vitamin D. These nutrients can be found in dairy products, leafy greens, fortified meals, and natural sunshine. Consuming them regularly might help maintain strong bones.

Protein is essential for maintaining healthy tissues and muscles. Supporting muscle maintenance and aiding recovery may be achieved by eating lean protein sources including poultry, fish, lentils, and tofu.

Cushing's illness is characterised by inflammation, which can be controlled by eating foods known for their anti-inflammatory properties. Anti-inflammatory foods include things like fruits, vegetables, whole grains, and healthy fats like those found in avocados and nuts.

Individuals with Cushing's disease should consult with a healthcare provider or qualified dietitian to create a diet plan that takes into account their unique requirements and medical conditions. To improve one's diet and health in general, they might offer tailored advice and assistance.

CHAPTER 4: RECOMMENDED FOODS FOR CUSHING'S DISEASE

People with Cushing's disease may benefit from include certain items in their diet. These foods can aid in general health maintenance, symptom control, and medication synergy. Examples are give below:

- Vitamins, minerals, and antioxidants may be found in fruits and vegetables, therefore it's important to eat a wide range of these foods. Fruits and vegetables with a lot of colour, such berries, citrus, leafy greens, broccoli, and bell peppers, are good choices.

- Go for whole grains like quinoa, brown rice, oats, and whole wheat bread. These are high in fibre and provide steady energy, two factors that contribute to better digestion and blood sugar control.

- Chicken, turkey, fish, beans, and tofu are all good sources of lean protein that you may add to your diet. These protein sources aid in the process of repairing and maintaining muscle tissue.

- Eat foods high in healthful fats, such avocados, nuts, seeds, and olive oil. These fats have been shown to enhance cardiovascular health and decrease inflammation.

- Dairy products, fortified soy and nut milks, dark green vegetables, and almonds are all good sources of calcium. Because of the higher risk of osteoporosis in Cushing's illness, calcium supplementation is recommended.

It is best to engage with a healthcare provider or trained dietitian to create a customised meal plan that takes into account food allergies, medicines, and general health objectives. They can help you improve your diet and overall health by giving you personalised advice and assistance. Before making any major dietary changes, it's important to talk to your healthcare providers.

Foods to Avoid or Limit in Cushing's Disease

Some foods should be avoided or consumed in moderation when dealing with Cushing's disease. High-sodium diets have been linked to water retention and hypertension.

When trying to limit sodium intake, it's best to cut back on processed meals like soups in a can, fast food, and salty snacks. These foods and drinks typically contain high levels of salt, which can disrupt the body's fluid balance and increase the risk of hypertension.

Individuals with Cushing's illness should also reduce their intake of added sugars. Weight gain, exacerbated insulin resistance, and metabolic imbalances are all possible outcomes of a diet heavy in sugary foods and beverages.

Fried and processed meals tend to be high in trans fats, which should be avoided. Individuals with Cushing's illness already have an increased risk of heart disease and inflammation, which can be further exacerbated by the consumption of these harmful fats.

The detrimental effects of alcohol on health are sufficient reason to restrict or abstain from drinking. Cushing's disease symptoms and problems can be made worse by alcohol use, which can throw off hormone balance, damage liver function, and cause weight gain.

Coffee, tea, and energy drinks are all sources of caffeine, which should be consumed in moderation. Caffeine can have a negative impact on hormone balance and sleep patterns, both of which are crucial in the management of Cushing's disease, although modest to moderate quantities can be tolerated.

Whole grains, fruits, and vegetables with a lower glycemic index should be substituted for high-glycemic index items such white bread, white rice, and sugary cereals. Eating these meals regularly can help maintain healthy blood sugar levels, increase feelings of fullness, and improve metabolic function.

In order to properly manage Cushing's disease, it is recommended to work with a healthcare expert or registered dietitian who specialises in endocrine diseases in order to receive personalised direction and assistance in developing a healthy, balanced food plan. They may provide you advice that is uniquely suited to you by taking into account things like your current medications, any health conditions, and dietary choices.

Meal Planning and Portion Control for Cushing's Disease

Meal planning and portion control are helpful for managing Cushing's disease and maintaining a healthy weight. A good food plan can help with blood sugar regulation, weight maintenance, and prevention of complications.

Preparing nutritious meals requires a focus on whole foods. Diversify your diet with fresh produce, lean meats, and whole grains. Vitamins, minerals, and antioxidants are abundant in these diets, whereas unnecessary carbohydrates and unhealthy fats are not.

Portion management is an effective tool for preventing overeating and maintaining a healthy weight. Eat meals that have the correct proportions of carbohydrates, protein, and fat. Use a food scale or measuring cups to ensure uniform portions.

Another helpful strategy is to eat multiple smaller meals instead of three large ones. This strategy can be useful for preventing blood sugar swings, keeping you alert for longer, and squelching the type of extreme hunger that can lead to binge eating.

In addition to planning meals and reducing portion sizes, paying attention to symptoms of hunger and fullness is crucial. Pay attention to your body's indications for when it's full, and stop eating before you feel stuffed. This strategy has the potential to promote a healthy relationship with food and reduce instances of overeating.

Be careful to stay well hydrated by drinking plenty of water throughout the day. Maintaining a healthy weight and maintaining proper body temperature are just two of the many health advantages of drinking enough water.

A qualified dietician who focuses on endocrine illnesses can help you create a tailored diet plan and learn to control your food consumption. Cushing's disease may be managed with their aid if you learn about your dietary alternatives, maintain track of your needs, and establish a sustainable eating pattern.

Cooking Methods and Preparation Techniques

Healthy, low-fat cooking methods that preserve the nutritional content of meals while minimising the addition of bad fats and excessive calories are recommended for people with Cushing's disease.

Steaming is a highly suggested cooking method. Steaming vegetables, fish, or chicken keeps their nutrients intact and reduces the number of calories they contain. Vitamins, minerals, and antioxidants can be preserved by cooking at low temperatures with as little water as possible.

Grilling or broiling is another method you may use to prepare your food healthily. By using this technique, the fat may easily drain out, leaving you with a leaner and healthier meal. A delightful smokey flavour is added without any additional fats. Be careful not to burn or char the food, as this might cause the formation of toxins.

Foods prepared in these ways are safe for people with Cushing's disease. Dry heat from the oven is used to get this tasty and tender product. When marinating or basting, use very little oil or choose healthy oils like olive or avocado oil.

For fast and healthy dinners, try stir-frying with a touch of healthy oil, such olive or coconut. To keep the food's texture and nutrition, cook it quickly over high heat while stirring constantly.

Reducing the amount of harmful ingredients like salt and sugar used in cooking is vital. Use herbs, spices, and other natural ingredients to boost the flavour instead. Without sacrificing flavour, this may give dimension to your dishes.

Fruits and vegetables, especially when eaten fresh or very gently cooked, may be a great source of vital nutrients and enzymes. To get the most nutrients out of your food, try eating it raw, in a smoothie, or minimally heated.

You may achieve your health objectives while controlling Cushing's disease by incorporating these cooking methods and preparation skills into your daily routine. To keep your diet balanced and nutritious, remember to focus on whole, unprocessed products and pay attention to serving quantities.

Healthier Cooking Methods

If you want to enhance your health and well-being, one of the first things you should do is start cooking using better ingredients and techniques. The nutritional value of foods can be preserved while their calorie and fat levels are reduced when better cooking methods are used.

Steaming is a healthy alternative to other cooking processes. Steaming is a method of cooking that uses the moist heat of steam to cook food without damaging the contents' nutritional value or flavour. It's a great option for anyone trying to limit their fat consumption because it calls for almost no additional fat.

Grilling or broiling is another useful technique. In contrast to broiling, which utilises indirect heat from above, grilling employs direct heat from below. Both procedures result in a slimmer end product because they allow superfluous fats to drain away. Adding oils or fats isn't necessary to get that delightful smokey flavour when grilling or broiling meals.

Roasting and baking are two more methods of cooking that are said to be better for you. Dry heat is used to cook food in the oven, and in most cases, no added oils or fats are necessary. The natural flavours of foods may be amplified and their nutritional value preserved by baking and roasting.

Stir-frying, in which food is cooked rapidly in a tiny amount of oil at high heat, is a common culinary technique. It keeps flavours and minerals intact while using hardly little oil at all. Stir-frying may be a healthy and savoury cooking method if you use olive oil or coconut oil and a wide choice of colourful veggies.

Sautéing, in which food is cooked in a minimal amount of oil over medium-high heat, is another option. Using this technique, you can prepare food quickly without sacrificing flavour or texture. Use oils that are better for you, and limit how much you use in the process.

Cooking using these ways reduces the amount of bad fats and calories consumed without sacrificing flavour or nutrition. Choose fresh, high-quality ingredients and season them with herbs, spices, and natural flavours to create delicious meals. With some ingenuity, you may prepare satisfying and healthful meals that contribute to your well-being.

Individualized Diet Plans and Consultation

In order to effectively manage Cushing's disease and achieve optimal health, tailored food programmes and counselling are essential. Different people have different dietary requirements and health concerns, therefore it's best to get advice from a doctor or a trained dietitian who can tailor a diet to your unique needs.

Dietary recommendations for people with Cushing's disease are developed after a thorough evaluation of the person's medical history, current symptoms, medicines, and desired outcomes. They will think about things like diet, exercise, and maintaining a healthy weight, as well as how well one's bones and heart are doing.

The goal of the customised eating plan will likely be to provide enough nutrition through consumption of a wide range of foods. Weight management, including limiting caloric intake to prevent or treat obesity, may be helpful for patients with Cushing's disease. Focus will be placed on portion management and eating balanced meals that include all three macronutrients (carbs, proteins, and healthy fats).

Lean proteins like poultry, fish, tofu, or lentils may be recommended as part of a tailored nutrition plan to promote muscle health and recovery. Vitamins, minerals, and fibre may all be attained through a diet rich in fruits, vegetables, whole grains, and low-fat dairy products.

The doctor may also stress the need of limiting salt consumption in the context of controlling swelling and blood pressure. They could suggest cutting back on processed and quick meals as well as those heavy in added sugars, saturated and trans fats, and other inflammatory food groups.

The nutrition plan may also contain suggestions for improving bone health, such as increasing calcium and vitamin D consumption through food or supplements, and recommending optimal fluid intake.

Adjustments may be made, progress can be monitored, and any problems that arise during the diet transition can be addressed during the follow-up appointments. In order to aid people in making educated food choices and keeping up a healthy diet, it may be helpful to teach them how to read product labels, create good meal plans, and prepare nutritious meals.

Overall, individualised diet plans and counselling are helpful in controlling Cushing's disease since they cater to the individual's particular dietary demands while simultaneously enhancing health. For the best possible health results, it is essential to coordinate your nutrition plan with your healthcare providers.

CHAPTER 5: 100+ SUPERFOODS RECIPES FOR CUSHING'S DISEASE

BREAKFAST RECIPE SUGGESTIONS

Classic poached eggs

Ingredients

- 2 eggs

- 15 mL (1 tbsp) white vinegar

- 1 whole grain English muffin, split and toasted

- Pinch of ground pepper

Directions

1. Bring a saucepan of water just to the boil. If it starts to boil, reduce heat to simmer.

2. In a small bowl, crack an egg. Stir vinegar into boiling water.

3. Lower the bowl close to the water's surface and gently slip egg into the water. Repeat with remaining egg. Let eggs cook for about 3 minutes or until whites are set and yolks are soft. Leave in longer for a firmer poached egg. Using a slotted spoon, remove eggs, one at a time.

4. Place one egg on each muffin half and sprinkle with pepper to serve.

Egg and veggie scramble

Ingredients

- 6 eggs

- 60 mL (¼ cup) skim milk

- 1 mL (¼ tsp) ground black pepper

- 5 mL (1 tsp) vegetable oil

- 375 mL (1 ½ cups) mixed frozen or fresh vegetables (such as onions, bell peppers, mushrooms)

Directions

1. In a medium bowl, beat together eggs, milk and pepper with a fork. Set aside.

2. In a medium 25 cm (10 inch) non-stick skillet, heat oil over medium heat. Add mixed vegetables and cook for 2 to 3 minutes stirring often until tender. If vegetables release too much liquid, increase heat for the last minute until liquid evaporates.

3. Reduce heat to medium-low and pour egg mixture over the vegetables. Continue cooking, without stirring, for 3 minutes or until eggs start to set. Use a heatproof spatula or wooden spoon and gently push mixture towards the centre of the pan and fold over, forming large pieces.

4. Continue gently folding eggs until cooked through, about 3 to 5 more minutes. Remove from heat and serve immediately.

Baked cheese stratas

Ingredients

- 2 slices whole grain bread

- 375 mL (1 ½ cups) chopped cooked broccoli

- 125 mL (½ cup) shredded lower fat old Cheddar or Swiss cheese

- 60 mL (¼ cup) chopped cooked turkey

- 30 mL (2 tbsp) chopped fresh parsley

- 190 mL (¾ cup) skim milk

- 3 eggs

- 5 mL (1 tsp) Dijon mustard

- Pinch of ground black pepper

Directions

1. Preheat the oven to 190 °C (375 °F).

2. Cut bread into 1 cm (½ inch) cubes using a serrated knife and place in a large bowl. Mix in broccoli, cheese, turkey and parsley. Divide among four 250 mL (1 cup) ovenproof ramekins or bowls, and place on a small baking sheet.

3. In a separate bowl, whisk together milk, eggs, mustard, and pepper until well combined. Gently pour over top of each bread mixture; press down gently with a fork so the bread absorbs the egg mixture. Let stand for 15 minutes or alternatively, cover and refrigerate for up to 12 hours.

4. Bake in preheated oven for about 35 minutes or until puffed and edges are golden, and a knife inserted in centre comes out clean. Use a digital food thermometer to check that the eggs have reached an internal temperature of 74°C (165°F).

Egg wrap with vegetables

Ingredients

- 1 egg or 2 egg whites

- 30 mL (2 tbsp) diced red bell pepper

- 30 mL (2 tbsp) grated zucchini or carrot

- Pinch of ground black pepper

- 1 small whole grain flour tortilla

- 15 mL (1 tbsp) grated lower fat old Cheddar or Swiss cheese

Directions

1. In a small bowl, beat together egg, red pepper, zucchini and pepper with a fork.

2. Spray a small non-stick skillet with cooking spray and place on medium heat. Pour egg mixture into the pan, swirling it to coat evenly. Let cook for about 2 minutes or until edge is light golden.

3. Using a spatula, lift around edges, flip egg over, and cook for another 30 seconds or until set and light golden.

4. Slide egg onto flour tortilla and sprinkle with cheese. Roll up and enjoy!

Carrot potato pancakes

Ingredients

- 4 eggs

- 500 mL (2 cups) finely grated carrot

- 500 mL (2 cups) finely grated potato

- 15 mL (1 tbsp) finely grated onion

- 30 mL (2 tbsp) whole wheat flour

- 2 mL (½ tsp) baking powder

Directions

1. Beat eggs in a large bowl. Stir in carrot, potato, onion, flour, and baking powder. Mix well.

2. Spray griddle or non-stick skillet lightly with cooking spray. Heat over medium heat. Using 125 mL (½ cup) measuring cup, pour batter onto hot griddle. Cook for about 2 minutes or until light golden brown. Flip over and cook for another minute or until light golden brown. Repeat with remaining batter.

Caprese muffin-tin frittatas

Ingredients

• 6 eggs

• 85 mL (⅓ cup) skim milk or unsweetened fortified plant-based beverages

• 2 mL (½ tsp) salt

• 2 mL (½ tsp) pepper

• 2 tomatoes, diced

• 5 mL (1 tsp) dried basil

• 125 mL (½ cup) grated lower fat mozzarella cheese

Directions

1. Preheat the oven to 200 °C (400 °F). Lightly spray or paper-line 6 muffin tins.

2. In a large bowl, whisk together eggs, milk, salt and pepper. Add tomatoes and basil and whisk well.

3. Using a 125 mL (½ cup) measuring cup, scoop batter into muffin tins until divided evenly. Add 15 mL (1 tbsp) of grated cheese on top of each frittata.

4. Cook frittatas in the oven for about 15 minutes. Use a digital food thermometer to check that the eggs have reached an internal temperature of 74 °C (165 °F).

5. Let cool for 3 to 5 minutes before removing from muffin tins.

Couscous and egg wraps

Ingredients

- 125 mL (½ cup) whole grain couscous

- 1 clove garlic, minced

- 2 mL (½ tsp) dried thyme or Italian herb seasoning

- 175 mL (¾ cup) lower sodium vegetable or chicken broth

- 60 mL (¼ cup) each grated carrot and zucchini or diced bell pepper

- 3 hard cooked eggs, peeled

- 85 mL (⅓ cup) 0% fat plain Greek yogurt

- 125 mL (½ cup) quartered grape tomatoes

- 60 mL (¼ cup) crumbled light feta cheese

- 45 mL (3 tbsp) chopped fresh basil or parsley

- 1 mL (¼ tsp) fresh ground pepper

- 4 small whole grain flour tortillas

Directions

1. Place couscous in a bowl with garlic and thyme. Bring broth to a boil and pour over couscous. Stir in carrot and zucchini; cover and let stand for 5 minutes.

2. Meanwhile, in another bowl, mash eggs with a fork and stir in yogurt, tomatoes,

feta, basil and pepper. Add couscous mixture and stir to combine.

3. Divide among the tortillas and roll up to enjoy.

Savoury broccoli and cheese muffins

Ingredients

- 125 mL (½ cup) all purpose flour

- 125 ml (½ cup) whole wheat flour

- 125 mL (½ cup) fine cornmeal

- 85 mL (⅓ cup) ground flax seed or wheat germ

- 5 mL (1 tsp) baking powder

- 5 mL (1 tsp) baking soda

- 2 mL (½ tsp) garlic powder

- 2 mL (½ tsp) paprika

- 1 mL (¼ tsp) cayenne

- 250 mL (1 cup) 0% plain Greek yogurt

- 85 mL (⅓ cup) skim milk

- 1 egg

- 30 mL (2 tbsp) vegetable oil

- 375 mL (1 ½ cups) chopped fresh or frozen broccoli florets

- 190 mL (¾ cup) shredded lower fat old Cheddar cheese

Directions

1. Preheat the oven to 200 °C (400 °F) and lightly spray or paper-line muffin pan.

2. In a large bowl, whisk together all purpose flour, whole wheat flour, cornmeal, ground flax, baking powder, baking soda, garlic powder, paprika and cayenne; set aside.

3. In a separate bowl, whisk together yogurt, milk, egg and oil. Pour over flour mixture and stir to combine. Stir in broccoli and cheese. (The batter will be thick.)

4. Scoop batter into muffin pan and bake for about 12 minutes or until golden and firm to the touch. Let cool slightly before removing from pan.

Multigrain congee with shiitake, ginger and scallion

Ingredients

- 6 dried shiitake mushrooms

- 60 mL (¼ cup) uncooked wheat berries, rinsed in cold water

- 85 mL (⅓ cup) uncooked Calrose, jasmine or other medium grain white rice, rinsed in cold water

- 30 mL (2 tbsp) uncooked black rice or other whole grain rice, rinsed in cold water

- 60 mL (¼ cup) uncooked millet or sorghum

- 1 ¾ L (7 cups) cold water, divided

- 6 pieces scallion, roots removed and thinly sliced

- 30 mL (2 tbsp) fresh ginger, peeled and thinly sliced

- 5 mL (1 tsp) sesame oil, toasted

- 15 mL (1 tbsp) lower sodium soy sauce

- Salt and white pepper to taste

Directions

1. Soak shiitake mushrooms in 250 mL (1 cup) cold water for 12 hours in the refrigerator. Remove any tough stems and cut pre-soaked mushrooms into ½ cm (¼ inch) slices. Reserve soaking liquid.

2. In a large pot, bring shiitakes, soaking liquid, wheat berries, white rice, black rice,

millet, and cold water to a simmer over medium heat.

3. Cover congee and cook for 1 hour and 15 minutes, stirring every 15 minutes to prevent grains from sticking to the bottom of the pot as they become softer. The congee is ready to eat when grains have broken down and mixture is creamy.

4. Serve hot congee in bowls. Garnish each bowl with scallions, ginger, toasted sesame oil, and lower sodium soy sauce. Season with salt and white pepper to taste.

Strawberry pancakes

Ingredients

- 250 mL (1 cup) whole wheat flour

- 125 mL (½ cup) all purpose flour

- 30 mL (2 tbsp) granulated sugar

- 10 mL (2 tsp) baking powder

- Pinch ground cinnamon

- 375 mL (1 ½ cups) skim milk

- 1 egg

- 30 mL (2 tbsp) vegetable oil

- 10 mL (2 tsp) vanilla

- 250 mL (1 cup) diced fresh strawberries

Directions

1. Preheat oven at 120 °C (250 °F).

2. In a large bowl, whisk together whole wheat flour, all purpose flour, sugar, baking powder, and cinnamon.

3. In a separate bowl, whisk together milk, egg, oil, and vanilla. Pour over flour mixture and stir to combine. Stir in strawberries.

4. Lightly spray a non-stick pan or griddle with cooking spray and heat over medium heat. Using a 60 mL (¼ cup) measuring cup, pour batter onto hot pan. Cook for about 2 minutes or until bubbles start to appear on top. Flip over and cook for another minute or until light golden brown. Repeat with remaining batter. Place pancakes on a baking sheet and keep warm in a preheated oven.

Apple pie breakfast bowl

Ingredients

- 125 mL (½ cup) uncooked quinoa

- 250 mL (1 cup) unsweetened fortified plant-based beverage or lower fat milk

- 125 mL (½ cup) water

- 1 mL (¼ tsp) ground cinnamon

- ½ mL (⅛ tsp) ground nutmeg

- 20 mL (1 ½ tbsp) honey

- 1 apple, finely diced

- 5 mL (1 tsp) vanilla extract

- 60 mL (¼ cup) raisin

Directions

1. Thoroughly rinse quinoa using a strainer and place in a small pot with a tight-fitting lid.

2. Stir in milk, water, cinnamon, nutmeg, honey, and apple.

3. Bring to a boil and reduce to a simmer. Cover and cook for 10 minutes or until all the liquid is absorbed.

4. Stir in vanilla extract and top with raisins.

Tofu and berry sheet tart

Ingredients

- 375 mL (1 ½ cups) frozen mixed berries

- 30 mL (2 tbsp) cornstarch

- 1 package (300 g/10.5 oz) soft tofu

- 15 mL (1 tbsp) honey

- 5 mL (1 tsp) vanilla extract

- 1 sheet (225 g/8 oz) puff pastry, thawed

- 125 mL (½ cup) unsalted pumpkin seeds

Directions

1. Preheat the oven to 190 °C (375 °F) and line a baking sheet with parchment paper.

2. In a small bowl, mix berries and cornstarch together. Set aside.

3. Drain excess liquid from the tofu. In a separate bowl, mash until smooth and stir in honey and vanilla extract.

4. Roll out the puff pastry into roughly a 23x30 cm (9x12 inch) rectangle. Place onto the baking sheet. Spread tofu on top, making sure to leave a 2.5 cm (1 inch) border. Spoon mixed berries onto tofu.

5. Bake for 25 to 30 minutes, until the edges are golden brown and fruits bubble.

6. Remove from the oven and top with pumpkin seeds or your family's favorite nuts or seeds.

Fruit salad

Ingredients

- 2 apples, cored and chopped

- 2 oranges, peeled and chopped

- ½ cantaloupe, seeded and chopped

- 2 pears, cored and chopped

- 30 mL (2 tbsp) lime juice (about 1 lime)

Directions

1. Add apples, oranges, cantaloupe and pears to a bowl. Squeeze lime juice over fruit. Toss together and serve immediately or chill until ready to eat.

Berry brunch bake

Ingredients

- 125 mL (½ cup) whole wheat flour

- 125 mL (½ cup) all-purpose flour

- 310 mL (1 ¼ cups) lower fat milk or unsweetened fortified plant-based beverage

- 4 eggs

- 5 mL (1 tsp) vanilla extract

- 20 mL (1 ½ tbsp) honey

- 10 mL (2 tsp) non-hydrogenated margarine

- 45 mL (3 tbsp) vegetable oil

- 375 mL (1 ½ cups) frozen berries

- 125 mL (½ cup) almonds, slivered or chopped

Directions

1. Preheat the oven to 250 °C (475 °F).

2. In a blender, place whole wheat flour, all-purpose flour, milk, eggs, vanilla, and honey. Blend on high until smooth.

3. In a 28x33 cm (11x13 inch) baking dish, put margarine and oil and place into pre-heated oven for 3 minutes, until margarine is melted.

4. Carefully and quickly, remove the hot baking dish from the oven and pour batter into the hot dish. Scatter top with berries and return to the oven immediately.

5. Bake for 20 minutes or until the batter is puffed and an inserted toothpick comes out clean.

6. Top with almonds and enjoy!

Fruit and yogurt granola parfaits

Ingredients

- 250 mL (1 cup) steel cut oats

- 250 mL (1 cup) large flake oats

- 165 mL (⅔ cup) slivered almonds

- 85 mL (⅓ cup) wheat germ

- 60 mL (¼ cup) flaxseed meal

- 45 mL (3 tbsp) pure maple syrup

- 15 mL (1 tbsp) vanilla

- 30 mL (2 tbsp) vegetable oil

- 1 L (4 cups) 0% plain Greek yogurt

- 750 mL (3 cups) fresh or frozen berries, such as raspberries, blueberries or blackberries

Directions

1. Preheat the oven to 180 °C (350 °F).

2. On a large baking sheet, spread steel-cut oats, large flake oats, almonds, wheat germ and flaxseed meal in single layer. Bake in preheated oven, stirring a couple of times, for about 15 minutes or until light golden. Scrape into a bowl.

3. In a small bowl, whisk together maple syrup, vanilla and oil. Pour over oat mixture and stir to coat evenly. Spread mixture onto baking sheet and return to oven for about 15 minutes or until golden brown, stirring at least twice. Let cool completely.

4. When ready to serve, divide half the granola among 10 small glasses or parfait dishes. Divide yogurt among glasses and sprinkle with some fruit. Top with remaining granola and fruit and enjoy. Alternatively, cover and refrigerate for up to a day.

Sweet zucchini muffins

Ingredients

- 60 mL (¼ cup) vegetable oil

- 165 mL (⅔ cup) packed brown sugar

- 1 egg

- 1 very ripe banana, mashed (about 125 mL/½ cup)

- 1 zucchini, grated

- 5 mL (1tsp) ground cinnamon

- 125 mL (½ cup) 0% plain Greek yogurt

- 5 mL (1 tsp) vanilla extract

- 250 mL (1 cup) all purpose flour with added bran or all purpose flour

- 190 mL (¾ cup) wheat bran

- 60 mL (¼ cup) wheat germ

- 5 mL (1 tsp) baking powder

- 2 mL (½ tsp) baking soda

- 125 mL (½ cup) raisins or dried cranberries or dried blueberries

Directions

1. Preheat the oven to 200 °C (400 °F) and lightly spray or paper-line muffin pan.

2. In a large bowl, whisk together oil, sugar and egg. Add banana, zucchini and cinnamon; stir in yogurt and vanilla.

3. In another bowl, whisk together flour, wheat bran and germ, baking powder and soda. Add flour mixture to banana mixture and stir until just moistened. Stir in raisins.

4. Divide evenly in muffin pan and bake for about 18 minutes or until light golden and firm to the touch. Let cool slightly before enjoying.

Cornmeal porridge with fruit preserve

Ingredients

- 1 L (4 cups) maple water

- 500 mL (2 cups) yellow cornmeal, medium grind

- 1 L (4 cups) of fresh or frozen berries

- 250 ml (1 cup) of water

- 30 mL (2 tbsp) of sugar

- 20 mL (4 tsp) maple syrup

Directions

1. In a pan, bring maple water to a boil then reduce to a simmer.

2. Stir in cornmeal and fold gently (do not stop or the mixture will clump together). Remove from heat after 8 minutes.

3. Prepare fruit preserve: Mix berries, water, and sugar in a pot. Simmer for 15 minutes, until the mixture has reduced by half.

4. Divide cornmeal into 4 bowls. Top off with fruit preserve and maple syrup. Serve with berries.

Chocolate berry overnight oats

Ingredients

- 335 mL (1 ⅓ cups) rolled oats

- 250 mL (1 cup) skim milk or unsweetened fortified plant-based beverages

- 85 mL (⅓ cup) 0% plain Greek yogurt

- 1 ripe banana, mashed (about 125 mL/½ cup)

- 20 mL (4 tsp) maple syrup or brown sugar

- 15 mL (1 tbsp) cocoa powder

- 250 mL (1 cup) fresh or frozen raspberries

Directions

1. In a medium bowl, whisk together all **ingredients** except for raspberries. Spoon equally into 4 small jars or airtight containers.

2. Refrigerate for at least 4 hours, preferably overnight, before eating.

3. When ready to serve, top with raspberries.

Banana walnut loaf

Ingredients

- 2 eggs

- 85 mL (⅓ cup) maple syrup

- 5 mL (1 tsp) vanilla extract

- 125 mL (½ cup) vegetable oil

- 3 bananas, mashed

- 250 mL (1 cup) whole wheat flour

- 190 mL (¾ cup) all-purpose flour

- 5 mL (1 tsp) baking soda

- 5 mL (1 tsp) cinnamon

- 1 mL (¼ tsp) salt

- 250 ml (1 cup) unsalted walnuts, toasted and chopped

Directions

1. Preheat the oven to 175 °C (350 °F) and grease a loaf pan or line with parchment paper.

2. In a large bowl, mix eggs, maple syrup, vanilla extract, and oil together. Stir in mashed bananas and set aside.

3. In a separate bowl, mix flour, baking soda, cinnamon, and salt.

4. Add dry **ingredients** to wet ones and mix until just combined. Do not overmix.

5. Fold in toasted walnuts.

6. Pour batter into the loaf pan. Bake for 50 to 55 minutes, until an inserted toothpick comes out clean.

Apple pie oatmeal

Ingredients

- 250 mL (1 cup) water

- 625 mL (2 ½ cups) skim milk

- 335 mL (1 ⅓ cups) large flake oats

- 85 mL (⅓ cup) wheat germ

- 30 mL (2 tbsp) packed brown sugar

- 2 mL (½ tsp) pumpkin pie spice or ground cinnamon

- 1 apple, cored and diced

- 30 mL (2 tbsp) dried cranberries (optional)

Directions

1. In a large saucepan, bring water and milk to a gentle boil over medium-high heat. Stir in oats and wheat germ. Reduce heat to medium-low and stir in sugar and pumpkin pie spice. Cook, stirring for about 12 minutes or until almost thickened.

2. Remove from heat and stir in apple and cranberries, if using. Cover and let stand for 5 minutes before serving.

LUNCH RECIPE SUGGESTIONS

Cheesy broccoli toast

Ingredients

- 500 mL (2 cups) frozen broccoli

- 2 slices whole grain bread

- 1 mL (¼ tsp) red pepper flakes

- 2 mL (½ tsp) garlic powder

- 2 slices whole grain bread

- 60 mL (¼ cup) shredded lower fat cheddar cheese

Directions

1. Preheat oven to 200 °C (400 °F).

2. Place frozen broccoli in a microwaveable bowl, cover with a plate and microwave on high for approximately 5 minutes. Allow to cool slightly then roughly mash with a fork. Add pepper flakes and garlic.

3. Lightly toast bread in oven or toaster. Place toast on a baking tray. Layer mashed broccoli mixture on each slice and evenly sprinkle the grated cheddar cheese over each slice.

4. Bake in the oven until cheese is melted and golden, approximately 5 minutes.

Quinoa and vegetable casserole

Ingredients

• 10 mL (2 tsp) extra virgin olive oil

• 1 leek, white and light green part only, thinly sliced

• 3 cloves garlic, minced

• 1 red, orange or yellow bell pepper, diced

• 10 mL (2 tsp) Italian herb seasoning

• 250 mL (1 cup) quinoa, rinsed

• 500 mL (2 cups) broccoli florets

• 440 mL (1 ¾ cups) sodium-reduced vegetable broth

- 250 mL (1 cup) frozen corn kernels

- 15 mL (1 tbsp) chopped fresh parsley

- 190 mL (¾ cup) shredded lower fat old Cheddar cheese

Directions

1. In a large non-stick skillet, heat oil over medium heat and cook leek, garlic, red pepper and Italian herb seasoning for 5 minutes or until starting to soften.

2. Stir in quinoa, broccoli and vegetable broth. Bring to a boil; reduce heat to low and cover and cook for about 15 minutes or until quinoa is tender. Stir in corn and parsley, and cook for 5 minutes.

3. Spoon mixture into small casserole dish and sprinkle with cheese.

4. Bake in preheated 200 °C (400 °F) oven for about 10 minutes or until cheese is melted.

Turkey stir-fry

Ingredients

- 30 mL (2 tbsp) canola oil, divided

- 500 g (1 lb) ground turkey

- Pinch ground cumin

- 1 carrot, thinly sliced

- 1 onion, thinly sliced

- Pinch cayenne

- ¼ head cabbage, shredded

- 2 cloves garlic, chopped

- 10 mL (2 tsp) lower sodium soy sauce

- 15 mL (1 tbsp) ketchup

- 125 mL (½ cup) frozen green beans

- 125 mL (½ cup) frozen corn

- Salt and pepper to taste

Directions

1. In a large pan, heat 15 mL (1 tbsp) oil over medium heat. Add turkey and cumin and cook for 6 to 8 minutes, stirring to break up the meat as it browns. Use a digital food thermometer to check that the turkey has reached an internal temperature of 74 °C (165 °F). Set turkey aside in a plate.

2. Add remaining oil, carrot and onion. Cook for 2 minutes.

3. Add cayenne, cabbage and garlic and continue to cook for 5 minutes or until soft.

4. Add soy sauce, ketchup, green beans, and corn and return cooked turkey to the pan. Stir well. Cook for 5 minutes.

Spaghetti and turkey meatballs

Ingredients

• 1 pkg (450 g) lean ground turkey

• 45 mL (3 tbsp) seasoned whole grain breadcrumbs

- 90 mL (6 tbsp) freshly grated Parmesan cheese, divided

- 30 mL (2 tbsp) chopped fresh parsley

- 1 mL (¼ tsp) ground pepper

- 1 can (796 mL/28 oz) no salt added tomatoes, pureed

- 1 carrot, grated

- 1 small onion, finely chopped

- 2 cloves garlic, minced

- 2 sprigs of fresh basil

- 1 mL (¼ tsp) hot pepper flakes

- 1 pkg (375 g) whole grain spaghetti

Directions

1. Preheat oven to 180°C (350 °F).

2. In a large bowl, combine turkey, breadcrumbs, 45 mL (3 tbsp) of the cheese, parsley and pepper. Using a 15 mL (1 tbsp) measuring spoon, roll turkey mixture into meatballs and place on parchment paper lined baking sheet. Repeat with remaining mixture. Makes 24 meatballs. Bake for 10 minutes. Use a digital food thermometer to check that meatballs have reached an internal temperature of 74°C (165°F). Remove from oven.

3. Meanwhile, in a saucepan, bring pureed tomatoes, carrot, onion, garlic, basil and hot pepper flakes to a simmer. Add meatballs; cover saucepan slightly and simmer for about 30 minutes or until thickened.

4. In a pot of boiling water, cook spaghetti for about 10 minutes or until tender but firm. Drain well and return to pot. Toss with sauce and meatballs until well coated. Sprinkle with remaining cheese to serve.

Spaghetti squash method

Looking for a creative way to increase your vegetable intake? Swap out the pasta for spaghetti squash. Here are a few ways you can cook it.

1. Start by cutting the squash in half and scooping out the seeds.

2. Place the squash cut-side down in a baking dish. Make sure the dish is microwave or oven-safe, depending on how you plan to cook it.

3. Add about 2.5 cm (1 inch) of water to the baking dish.

4. Choose your method of cooking the squash. You can:

o microwave it for about 10 minutes or until soft

o roast it in the oven covered with aluminum foil in a baking dish. Cook at 200°C (400°F) for 30 to 45 minutes or until soft

5. Make the squash noodles once squash is cool enough to handle. Use a fork to pull the squash strands away from the rind. Toss the squash noodles in with the sauce and meatballs until well-coated.

6. Serve immediately or store in the fridge for 3 to 4 days or in the freezer for 2 to 3 months.

Chicken and bean quesadillas

Ingredients

- 15 mL (1 tbsp) vegetable oil

- 454 g (1 lb) ground chicken

- 15 mL (1 tbsp) chili powder

- 5 mL (1 tsp) cumin

- 20 mL (1 ½ tbsp) onion powder

- 20 mL (1 ½ tbsp) garlic powder

- 1 bell pepper, diced

- 375 mL (1 ½ cups) water

- 1 can (540 mL/19 oz) lower sodium black beans, drained and rinsed

- 250 mL (1 cup) frozen corn

- 30 mL (2 tbsp) lemon juice (about 1 lemon)

- 2 tomatoes, diced

To assemble:

- 10 small whole wheat tortillas

- 335 mL (1 ⅓ cups) shredded lower fat mozzarella cheese

Directions

1. Preheat the oven to 190 °C (375 °F) and line a baking sheet with aluminum foil.

2. In a large pan, heat vegetable oil over medium-high heat. Add chicken, chili powder, cumin, onion powder, and garlic powder. Stir frequently to prevent spices from burning until chicken is browned.

3. Stir in peppers and cook for 3 minutes. Add water and simmer until the water is reduced by ⅔. Use a digital food thermometer to check that the chicken has reached an internal temperature of 74 °C (165 °F).

4. Remove from heat and stir in black beans, corn, lemon juice, and tomatoes.

5. Place tortillas onto the baking sheet. On each tortilla, spread 125 mL (½ cup) of filling on half of the tortilla. Sprinkle with 30 mL (2 tbsp) of cheese and fold over in half.

6. Bake in the oven for 7 minutes until cheese is melted and tortilla is crisp.

Tuna salad wraps

Ingredients

- 1 can (120 g drained weight) light flaked tuna in water, drained

- 15 mL (1 tbsp) mayonnaise

- 5 mL (1 tsp) yellow mustard

- 5 mL (1 tsp) lemon juice

- 1 celery stalk, finely chopped

- 60 mL (¼ cup) green pepper, finely chopped

- 2 mL (½ tsp) black pepper

- 2 leaves romaine lettuce, washed and dried

- 2 whole grain tortillas

Directions

1. In a medium bowl, use a fork to combine tuna, mayonnaise, mustard and lemon.

2. Add celery, green pepper and black pepper to the tuna mixture and mix until well distributed.

3. Place 1 lettuce leaf on each tortilla.

4. Scoop half of the tuna mixture onto each wrap and roll up.

Moose stew

Ingredients

- 10 mL (2 tsp) vegetable oil

- 575 g (1 ¼ lb) moose, cubed

- 1 onion, cut into large chunks

- 3 celery stalks, chopped

- 5 carrots, peeled and chopped

- 1 L (4 cups) no salt added beef broth

- 5 yellow fleshed potatoes, peeled and diced

- 750 mL (3 cups) frozen mixed vegetables

- 2 mL (½ tsp) dried parsley

- 2 mL (½ tsp) dried thyme

- 4 bay leaves, dried

- 5 mL (1 tsp) pepper

Directions

1. In a large shallow saucepan or Dutch oven, heat oil over medium heat. Brown the moose meat and put aside.

2. Add the onions to the saucepan and cook for 2 to 3 minutes. Add the celery and carrots. Cook about 7 to 8 minutes, stirring frequently.

3. Add the moose meat and stir. Add in broth, potatoes, frozen vegetables, parsley, thyme, bay leaves and pepper and stir. Cover, lower heat and simmer for 2 hours. Use a digital food thermometer to check that the moose has reached an internal temperature of 74 °C (165 °F).

4. Remove whole bay leaves before serving.

Chicken and spring vegetable soup

Ingredients

- 1 ¼ L (5 cups) water

- 1 onion, sliced

- 2 mL (½ tsp) whole black peppercorns

- 2 dried bay leaves

- 15 mL (1 tbsp) lemon juice

- 2 boneless skinless chicken breasts (about 225 g/½ lb)

- ¼ head cabbage, thinly sliced

- 1 head broccoli, cut into small florets

- 1 carrot, thinly sliced

- 125 mL (½ cup) sliced mushrooms

- Salt to taste

Directions

1. In a medium pot with a lid, bring water to a boil. Add onion, peppercorns, bay leaves, and lemon juice. Reduce heat to low.

2. Add chicken and partially cover with lid. Poach chicken for 5 to 7 minutes, turning over once to cook evenly on both sides.

3. Using a slotted spoon, remove bay leaves and peppercorns and discard. Add cabbage, broccoli, carrot, and mushrooms.

4. Cover and simmer for 10 minutes. Use a digital food thermometer to check that chicken has reached an internal temperature of 74 °C (165 °F).

5. Slice chicken and return to the pot. Gently reheat on low heat for 4 minutes. Serve hot and season with salt to taste.

Shakshouka (poached eggs recipe)

Ingredients

- 1 yellow onion, diced

- 1 bell pepper, diced

- 4 cloves garlic, minced

- 796 mL (28 oz) can of no salt added diced tomatoes

- 5 mL (1 tsp) cumin

- 10 mL (2 tsp) paprika

- 2.5 mL (½ tsp) ground coriander

- 1.25 mL (¼ tsp) red pepper flakes

- 4 eggs

• Optional topping: parsley

Directions

1. Preheat the oven to 190°C (375°F).

2. Lightly coat a large oven-safe skillet with cooking spray or oil and heat over medium-high heat. Add diced onions and cook for 3 minutes, stirring frequently. Add bell pepper and garlic and continue to cook for 2 minutes.

3. Add canned tomatoes and all of the spices to the skillet and bring to a boil. Reduce the heat to medium-low and simmer for 10 minutes.

4. In a small bowl, crack one egg. Using a small spoon, move the simmering tomato mixture to create a small hole for the egg.

Pour the egg into the hole. Repeat until all eggs are in the skillet.

5. Turn off the heat and move the skillet from the stovetop to the preheated oven. Cook for 10-15 minutes until eggs are set but still jiggle in the centre when you move the skillet. They will continue to cook once removed from the oven.

6. Remove the skillet from the oven. Add a handful of chopped parsley, if desired, and serve.

Lentil nuggets

Ingredients

- 1 can (540 mL/19 oz) lentils, drained and rinsed

- 60 mL (¼ cup) rolled oats

- 30 mL (2 tbsp) lemon juice (about 1 lemon)

- 10 mL (2 tsp) dried basil

- 10 mL (2 tsp) cumin

- 5 mL (1 tsp) garlic powder

- 15 mL (1 tbsp) olive oil

Directions

1. In a blender or food processor, place all **ingredients** (except for olive oil) and blend until smooth.

2. Form mini patties with your hands by rolling about 15 mL (1 tbsp) of the mixture and then molding into the shape of little disks (or any other shape you like). Place patties on a plate.

3. In a large skillet, heat olive oil over medium-high heat. Gently transfer the nuggets to the skillet and pan-fry for about 2 to 3 minutes per side or until golden brown on both sides. Remove from skillet and allow to cool.

Toasted barley and wild rice salad

Ingredients

- 125 mL (½ cup) each pot barley and wild rice

- 250 mL (1 cup) lower sodium vegetable or chicken broth

- 250 mL (1 cup) water

- 1 orange or yellow bell pepper, chopped

- 1 zucchini, chopped

- 1 tomato, diced

- 30 mL (2 tbsp) cider or white wine vinegar

- 15 mL (1 tbsp) Dijon mustard

- 10 mL (2 tsp) vegetable oil

- 1 small clove garlic, finely grated

- Pinch of ground pepper

- 375 mL (1 ½ cups) chopped cooked turkey or chicken (about 180 g/6 oz)

- 60 mL (¼ cup) each chopped fresh parsley and chives

Directions

1. In a saucepan, toast barley and wild rice over medium heat, stirring for 3 minutes. Add broth and water; bring to a boil. Reduce heat to a simmer, cover and cook for about 30 minutes or until barley and rice are tender but still chewy and firm. Remove from heat and let cool slightly.

2. In a large bowl, combine cooled barley-rice mixture with bell pepper, zucchini and tomato.

3. In a small bowl, whisk together vinegar, mustard, oil, garlic and pepper. Drizzle over top of barley-rice mixture and stir to coat. Stir in turkey, parsley and chives until well distributed.

Slow-cooker burrito bowls

Ingredients

• 2 boneless skinless chicken breasts (about 680 g/1 ½ lb)

- 375 mL (1 ½ cups) canned (no salt added) diced tomatoes

- 310 mL (1 ¼ cups) lower sodium chicken broth

- 10 mL (2 tsp) chili powder

- 5 mL (1 tsp) ground cumin

- 5 ml (1 tsp) garlic powder

- 1 can (540 mL/19 oz) black beans, drained and rinsed

- 250 mL (1 cup) uncooked brown rice

- 250 mL (1 cup) frozen or canned (no salt added) corn

- Optional toppings: lower fat shredded mozzarella, lower fat plain yogurt, lower sodium salsa, diced fresh avocado

Directions

1. Lightly spray inside of large slow cooker with cooking spray.

2. In a large slow cooker, combine the chicken, diced tomatoes (with juice), chicken broth, chili powder, cumin, and garlic powder. Make sure the chicken broth covers the chicken, adding more if needed. Cover and cook for 3 to 4 hours on the low setting.

3. Uncover and stir in the beans, brown rice, and corn. Cover and cook for another 3 to 4 hours on the low setting.

4. In the last hour of cooking, check the brown rice occasionally, stirring once or twice to make sure it cooks evenly and adding more chicken broth if the mixture seems dry. Cooking is done when the brown rice is tender.

5. Remove the chicken and place in a large bowl or cutting board. Use 2 forks to shred the chicken into bite-sized pieces. Transfer the chicken back to the slow cooker and mix.

6. Serve in individual bowls alongside optional toppings of choice.

Chickpea and vegetable couscous

Ingredients

• 375 mL (1 ½ cups) uncooked whole grain couscous

• 1 rutabaga cut into 2.5 cm (1 inch) cubes

• 4 carrots, cubed

• 4 parsnips, cubed

• 2 celery stalks, sliced

• 1 can (540 mL/19 oz) chickpeas, drained and rinsed

• 1 can (796 mL/28 oz) diced no salt added tomatoes

• 15 mL (1 tbsp) couscous spice (see tip)

- 2 bay leaves

- 3 zucchini sliced into thick rounds

Directions

1. Bring 375 mL (1 ½ cups) of water to a boil, then remove from heat. Add couscous and cover, letting it absorb water for about 5 minutes. Once this is done, little chefs can fluff it with a fork.

2. Place rutabaga, carrots, parsnips, celery and chickpeas into a large pot.

3. Crush tomatoes using a blender, and place in the pot with spices and bay leaves. Add about 400 mL (1 ⅔ cup) of water, or until vegetables are just covered.

4. Bring to a boil, then lower the heat and simmer gently for 20 minutes until vegetables are tender.

5. Then add zucchini and continue cooking for 10 minutes. During this time, cook couscous.

6. Once the vegetables are cooked, remove bay leaves and serve on a bed of cooked couscous.

Honey grilled salmon and asparagus

Ingredients

Marinade:

- 15 mL (1 tbsp) lower sodium soy sauce

- 10 mL (2 tsp) vegetable oil

- 10 mL (2 tsp) liquid honey

- 10 mL (2 tsp) packed brown sugar

- 5 mL (1 tsp) chopped fresh thyme or 2 mL (½ tsp) dried thyme leaves

- 1 mL (¼ tsp) ground pepper

Fish and asparagus:

- 4 salmon fillets (about 565 g/1¼ lb)

- 1 bunch fresh asparagus, trimmed

- ½ lemon

Directions

1. Prepare the marinade: In a small bowl, stir together soy sauce, oil, honey, sugar, thyme and black pepper.

2. Place salmon in a shallow dish. Pour marinade over top of salmon, spreading evenly. Cover and refrigerate for 15 to 30 minutes, turning once if possible.

3. Lightly spray asparagus with cooking spray and place on preheated and oiled grill on medium high heat. Grill, turning a couple of times until tender crisp. Add salmon fillets and grill for 5 minutes. Discard marinade. Turn salmon over and grill for about 5 minutes longer or until fish flakes easily when tested *. Serve with asparagus. Squeeze lemon over asparagus just prior to serving.

Chickpea "meatballs" and gnocchi bake

Ingredients

Tomato sauce:

- 30 mL (2 tbsp) vegetable oil

- 1 onion, chopped

- 3 cloves garlic, minced

- 1 can (796 mL/28 oz) diced tomatoes

- 4 mL (¾ tsp) dried oregano

- ½ package (150 g/5 oz) frozen spinach, defrosted

Chickpea and mushroom "meatballs":

• 1 package (225 g/8 oz) cremini mushrooms, chopped finely (about 375 mL/1 ½ cups)

• 30 mL (2 tbsp) vegetable oil

• 1 mL (¼ tsp) salt

• 1 can (540 mL/19 oz) chickpeas, drained and rinsed

• 4 mL (¾ tsp) dried oregano

• 5 mL (1 tsp) garlic powder

• 15 mL (1 tbsp) dried parsley

• 1 egg

To assemble:

- 1 package (500 g/18 oz) gnocchi

- 250 mL (1 cup) shredded mozzarella cheese

Directions

1. Preheat the oven to 190 °C (375 °F) and line a baking sheet with aluminum foil. Set aside.

2. Prepare the tomato sauce: In a medium saucepan, heat vegetable oil. Sauté onions and garlic for 2 to 3 minutes or until fragrant.

3. Stir in tomatoes and oregano. Bring to a simmer and cook for 20 minutes.

4. Using a hand blender, purée sauce and stir in defrosted spinach.

5. Prepare the "meatballs": In a small pan, sauté mushrooms in vegetable oil and salt over medium heat. Cook for 10 minutes or until all the water evaporates and mushrooms are dry. Allow to cool.

6. Place chickpeas on the baking sheet and roast in the preheated oven for 5 minutes. Remove from the oven, place in a bowl, and crush with a fork or potato masher. Add cooked mushrooms to the bowl with crushed chickpeas.

7. Once cooled, stir in oregano, garlic, parsley, and egg. Form into 12 "meatballs" and place on the baking sheet.

8. Bake for 15 minutes or until internal temperature reaches 74 °C (165 °F).

9. Boil gnocchi per package instructions and add to tomato sauce. Pour into an oven safe casserole and top with baked "meatballs" and cheese. Return to oven for 20 minutes or until cheese is melted.

Curried lentil and spinach fritters

Ingredients

- 125 mL (½ cup) uncooked red split lentils

- 125 mL (½ cup) spinach, chopped finely

- 1 egg

- 5 mL (1 tsp) curry powder

- 1 mL (¼ tsp) black pepper

- 15 mL (1 tbsp) onion powder

- 2 mL (½ tsp) garlic powder

- 2 mL (½ tsp) baking soda

- 125 mL (½ cup) lower fat yogurt

- 85 mL (⅓ cup) whole wheat flour

- 15 mL (1 tbsp) vegetable oil

Cucumber Dipping Sauce:

- ½ large cucumber

- 125 mL (½ cup) lower fat yogurt

- 1 mL (¼ tsp) cumin

- 1 mL (¼ tsp) chili powder

- Salt to taste

Directions

1. Rinse lentils well, drain and place in a large microwave safe bowl with 500 mL (2 cups) water. Cover and microwave for 4 to 5 minutes or until lentils have softened. Carefully drain any excess water and allow to cool.

2. Stir in spinach, egg, curry powder, black pepper, onion powder, garlic powder, baking soda, yogurt, and flour.

3. In a pan, add 5 mL (1 tsp) oil, swirl to cover pan, and heat over medium heat.

4. Pan fry 30 mL (2 tbsp) fritters for 2 minutes per side. Repeat until all batter is used.

5. For the dipping sauce, grate cucumber into a bowl and squeeze out all excess liquid.

Stir in yogurt, cumin, chili, and season with salt to taste.

Whitefish tacos

Ingredients

Filling:

• 30 mL (2 tbsp) extra virgin olive oil

• 30 mL (2 tbsp) lemon juice (about 1 lemon)

• 5 mL (1 tsp) ground cumin

• 625 mL (2 ½ cups) cooked flaky white fish (like cod)

Lettuce slaw:

- 125 mL (½ cup) 0% plain Greek yogurt

- 15 mL (1 tbsp) extra virgin olive oil

- 30 mL (2 tbsp) lime juice (about 1 lime)

- 5 mL (1 tsp) garlic powder

- ½ head of lettuce, chopped

- 5 mL (1 tsp) dried cilantro

- 8 small whole grain corn tortillas

- Salt and pepper to taste

- Optional toppings: avocado, corn, Pico de Gallo or salsa, lime wedges

Directions

1. In a medium bowl, whisk together 30 mL (2 tbsp) olive oil, lemon juice, and cumin.

2. Add cooked fish, flaking it apart and coating it in the dressing.

3. Meanwhile, in a large bowl, whisk Greek yogurt, 15 mL (1 tbsp) olive oil, lime juice, garlic powder. Stir in lettuce and cilantro. Season with salt and pepper to taste.

4. Assemble tacos: Serve fish over tortillas with lettuce slaw and toppings of choice!

Okroshka (cold summer soup)

Ingredients

- 1 boiled potato, cubed

- 3 hard-boiled eggs, cubed

- 1 large cucumber, halved, seeds removed and diced into small cubes

- 1 bunch radishes, thinly sliced (about 250 mL/1 cup)

- 1 bunch scallions, dark and light green parts, thinly sliced (about 250 mL/1 cup)

- 250 mL (1 cup) fresh dill, finely chopped

- 500 mL (2 cups) 1% kefir

- 45 mL (3 tbsp) of lemon juice (about 1 lemon)

- Salt to taste

Directions

1. Thinly slice radishes using a mandolin or sharp knife. Arrange slices in small stacks on

your cutting board. Thinly slice the stacks of radish to make thin matchsticks.

2. In a large bowl, combine boiled potato, hard cooked eggs, cucumber, radish, scallions, and dill. Pour kefir over mixture, add lemon juice and stir well to combine.

3. Refrigerate and serve when ready.

Minestrone soup

Ingredients

- 1.5 L (6 cups) no salt added vegetable broth

- 1 L (4 cups) chopped cabbage

- 750 mL (3 cups) carrots, diced

- 1 can (540 mL/19 oz) no salt added white kidney beans, drained and rinsed

- 1 can (796 mL/28 oz) no salt added diced tomatoes or diced tomatoes in puree

- 2 mL (½ tsp) garlic powder

Directions

1. In a large pot, bring vegetable broth to a boil.

2. Reduce heat to medium. Add chopped cabbage and diced carrots. Cover and simmer until vegetables are tender, about 35 minutes.

3. Stir in beans, tomatoes and garlic powder. Add pepper to taste. Cover and cook 5 minutes longer.

4. Serve in bowls.

Beef and bean burger

Ingredients

- 1 can (540 mL/19 oz) low sodium black beans, drained and rinsed

- 125 mL (½ cup) finely chopped onion

- 3 cloves garlic, minced

- 30 mL (2 tbsp) Dijon mustard

- 5 mL (1 tsp) ground cumin

- 7 mL (½ tbsp) paprika

- 2 mL (½ tsp) salt

- 1 mL (¼ tsp) black pepper

- 1 egg

- 454 g (1 lb) extra lean ground beef

Directions

1. Preheat the oven to 200 °C (400 °F) and line a baking sheet with aluminum foil.

2. In a large bowl, mash black beans with a fork or a potato masher.

3. To the same bowl, mix in onion, garlic, mustard, cumin, paprika, salt, pepper, and egg.

4. Add ground beef and mix thoroughly. Firmly form into 8 burger patties and place onto the baking sheet.

5. Bake for 15 to 17 minutes. Use a digital food thermometer to check that the burgers have reached an internal temperature of 74 °C (165 °F).

DINNER RECIPE SUGGESTIONS

Chicken and lima bean stew

Ingredients

- 30 mL (2 tbsp) vegetable oil

- 6 boneless, skinless chicken thighs (about 454 g/1 lb), diced in 5 cm/2 inch cubes

- 1 onion, diced

- 3 cloves garlic, chopped

- 5 mL (1 tsp) ground cumin

- 5 mL (1 tsp) ground cinnamon

- 2 mL (½ tsp) ground clove

- 5 mL (1 tsp) salt

- 2 mL (½ tsp) black pepper

- 3 carrots, thinly sliced

- 500 mL (2 cups) frozen butternut squash cubes

- 750 mL (3 cups) fresh spinach, chopped

- 60 mL (¼ cup) dried apricots, quartered

- 125 mL (½ cup) unsalted almonds, roughly chopped (optional)

- 500 mL (2 cups) lower sodium vegetable broth

- 1 can (540 mL/19 oz) lower sodium lima beans, drained and rinsed

Directions

1. In a large pan, heat vegetable oil over medium-high heat. Cook chicken for 2 to 3 minutes per side until browned.

2. Reduce heat to medium and add onion, garlic, cumin, cinnamon, clove, salt, and pepper. Sauté for 2 to 3 minutes or until onions have softened.

3. Add carrots, squash, spinach, dried apricots, and almonds. Stir well and add broth.

4. Cover and simmer for 20 minutes until the chicken is tender and sauce has reduced. Use a digital food thermometer to check that the chicken has reached an internal temperature of 74 °C (165 °F).

5. Stir in lima beans to warm through and remove from heat.

6. Enjoy with brown rice or quinoa.

Harira (Moroccan stew)

Ingredients

- 10 mL (2 tsp) vegetable oil

- 1 onion, diced

- 10 mL (2 tsp) ground cinnamon

- 10 mL (2 tsp) ground cumin

- 10 mL (2 tsp) ground coriander

- A pinch of chili flakes (optional)

- 2 cloves garlic, minced

- 1 large sweet potato, peeled and chopped in 1.5 cm (½ inch) pieces

- 375 mL (1 ½ cups) peas, frozen

- 1 can (796 mL/28 oz) no salt added tomatoes, crushed

- 750 mL (3 cups) no salt added vegetable broth

- 1 can (540 mL/19 oz) no salt added chickpeas, drained and rinsed

Directions

1. In a saucepan, heat oil over medium heat and cook onion for 3 minutes or until softened. Add cinnamon, cumin, coriander,

chili flakes (optional) and garlic and stir, cooking over low heat for about another 2 minutes.

2. Add sweet potatoes, frozen peas and tomatoes and stir to coat vegetables in spices and oil.

3. Add the vegetable broth. Bring to a boil, reduce heat and simmer until the sweet potatoes are tender (about 25 minutes).

4. Stir in the chickpeas and simmer another 5 minutes or until the sweet potatoes are soft with a fork.

Turkey and vegetable pita

Ingredients

- 85 mL (⅓ cup) 0% fat plain Greek yogurt

- 30 mL (2 tbsp) light mayonnaise

- 5 mL (1 tsp) Dijon or yellow mustard

- 1 mL (¼ tsp) of ground black pepper

- 375 mL (1 ½ cups) chopped cooked turkey breast meat (about 227 g /8 oz)

- 125 mL (½ cup) diced red or green bell pepper

- 60 mL (¼ cup) grated carrot

- 2 whole grain pita pockets

- 4 leaves Boston lettuce

- Quarter of a large cucumber, thinly sliced

Directions

1. In a large bowl, whisk together yogurt, mayonnaise, mustard and pepper. Stir in turkey, red pepper and carrot until coated well.

2. Cut pitas in half and open pockets. Tuck lettuce and cucumber slices into each half and spoon in turkey mixture.

Slow-cooked lasagna

Ingredients

- 225 g (½ lb) extra lean ground beef

- 1 onion, finely chopped

- 3 cloves garlic, minced

- 10 mL (2 tsp) dried oregano

- 1 mL (¼ tsp) hot pepper flakes

- 1 jar (700 mL) passata (strained crushed tomatoes)

- 250 mL (1 cup) water

- 10 whole grain lasagna noodles

- 1 tub (475 g) light ricotta cheese

- 1 container (142 g/5 oz) baby spinach, washed, chopped

- 60 mL (¼ cup) chopped fresh basil or parsley

- 30 mL (2 tbsp) grated Parmesan cheese

- 125 mL (½ cup) shredded part skim mozzarella

Directions

1. Lightly spray inside of slow cooker with cooking spray.

2. In a large non-stick skillet, brown beef breaking up with spoon. Scrape out beef into a colander and let drain. Wipe out skillet and return to medium heat; cook beef, onion, garlic, oregano and hot pepper flakes for 5 minutes or until softened. Add passata and water and remove from heat.

3. In a bowl, stir together ricotta cheese, spinach, basil and Parmesan cheese.

4. Spread some of the meat sauce over bottom of slow cooker. Lay lasagna noodles in a single layer, breaking as necessary to fit. Top with one quarter of the sauce and one third of the cheese mixture. Repeat layers twice ending with meat sauce on top. Cover and cook on Low for 6 to 8 hours or on High for 3 to 4 hours. About 15 minutes before serving lasagna, sprinkle mozzarella over top, cover and let cook on Low until melted.

Curried vegetable lentil stew

Ingredients

- 10 mL (2 tsp) vegetable oil

- 1 red onion, chopped

- 4 cloves garlic, minced

- 60 mL (¼ cup) chopped fresh cilantro, divided

- 15 mL (1 tbsp) minced fresh ginger or 5 mL (1 tsp) ground ginger

- 30 mL (2 tbsp) mild curry paste or powder

- 5 mL (1 tsp) garam masala

- 30 mL (2 tbsp) all purpose flour

- 625 mL (2 ½ cups) lower sodium vegetable broth

- 2 yellow fleshed potatoes, diced

- 1 red bell pepper, chopped

- 310 mL (2¼ cup) fresh or frozen green beans, chopped

- 1 can (540 mL/19 oz) lentils, drained and rinsed

Directions

1. In a large shallow saucepan or Dutch oven, heat oil over medium heat. Cook onion, garlic, half of the cilantro, ginger, curry paste and garam masala for about 3 minutes or until softened. Stir in flour until absorbed. Slowly pour in broth, stirring until combined.

2. Add potatoes, pepper, beans and lentils and bring to a simmer. Cover and cook, stirring often, for about 20 minutes or until potatoes are tender. Sprinkle with remaining cilantro before serving.

Simple breakfast soup

Ingredients

- 30 mL (2 tbsp) olive oil

- ½ yellow onion, finely chopped

- 2 garlic cloves, minced

- 2 celery stalks, small diced

- 2 carrots, peeled and small diced

- ½ bunch broccoli, including stems, trimmed and finely chopped (about 750 mL/3 cups)

- 1 can (540 mL/19 oz) no salt added chickpeas, drained and rinsed

- 1 L (4 cups) water

- 15 mL (1 tbsp) white miso

- 30 mL (2 tbsp) cold water

- Salt and pepper to taste

Directions

1. In a pot, heat oil over medium heat. Add onion, garlic, celery and carrot and cook for 6 to 8 minutes or until carrots are tender. Add broccoli and chickpeas and cook for 2 more minutes.

2. Add water and bring to a boil. Reduce heat and simmer for 10 minutes or until vegetables are tender. Remove from heat.

3. In a small bowl, whisk together miso and cold water, then stir into soup.

4. Let cool slightly before serving. Season with salt and pepper to taste.

Chickpea and vegetable curry

Ingredients

- 45 mL (3 tbsp) curry powder

- 420 mL (1 ½ cups + 3 tbsp) water, divided

- ½ yellow onion, cut in quarters

- 3 cloves garlic

- 1 stalk of celery

- 60 mL (¼ cup) diced green bell pepper

- 1 tomato, cut in half

- 5 mL (1 tsp) garam masala

- 2.5 mL (½ tsp) salt

- 1 can (540 mL/19 oz) no salt added chickpeas, drained and rinsed

- 500 mL (2 cups) cauliflower, cut in bite-sized pieces

- 250 mL (1 cup) frozen peas, thawed

Directions

1. In a small bowl, mix the curry powder with 45 mL (3 tbsp) water. Mix into a loose paste and set aside.

2. In a food processor, purée ¼ of the onion, the garlic, celery, green pepper, and ½ the tomato. It doesn't have to be completely smooth, but should be well incorporated.

3. Dice remaining onion and other ½ tomato.

4. Lightly coat a large non-stick pan with cooking spray or oil and heat over medium-high heat. Add curry paste and cook, about 30 seconds.

5. Add in vegetable purée, diced onion and tomato to the pot. Lower the heat to medium and sauté for 10 minutes, stirring frequently.

6. Add 375 mL (1 ½ cups) of water, garam masala and salt to the pot and allow the mixture to simmer on medium-low covered for 10 minutes. Stir occasionally.

7. Increase the heat to medium-high and add in chickpeas and cauliflower. Cook until cauliflower reaches desired level of

doneness. Add in peas at the very end just to warm them up.

Sweet potato curry

Ingredients

- 30 mL (2 tbsp) vegetable oil, divided

- 5 mL (1 tsp) black mustard seeds

- 3 whole dried red chilies

- 4 fresh or dried curry (neem) leaves

- 1 onion, finely diced

- 2 cloves garlic, finely chopped

- 3 sweet potatoes, peeled and chopped into a 1-inch dice

- 1 small handful fresh coriander, finely chopped (about 60 mL/¼ cup)

- Salt to taste

Directions

1. In a high-sided sauté pan, heat oil over high heat. Add mustard seeds, chilies, and curry leaves and sauté for 30 seconds to release flavours.

2. Add onions and sauté for 2 minutes or until just lightly browned. Add garlic and stir to combine. Sauté for another 3 minutes or until onions soften.

3. Add sweet potatoes and stir to combine and coat well. Reduce heat to medium and cook for 20 to 30 minutes or until tender.

4. Sprinkle coriander on top and serve.

Mapo tofu with chicken

Ingredients

- 45 mL (3 tbsp) sesame oil

- 5 mL (1 tsp) chili flakes

- 454 g (1 lb) ground chicken

- 15 mL (1 tbsp) chopped ginger

- 15 mL (1 tbsp) chopped garlic

- 15 mL (1 tbsp) tomato paste

- 45 mL (3 tbsp) lower sodium soy sauce

- 500 mL (2 cups) lower sodium vegetable broth

- 15 mL (1 tbsp) cornstarch

- 60 mL (¼ cup) water

- 1 package (400 g/14 oz) medium-firm tofu, cubed

- 60 mL (¼ cup) sliced green onion

Directions

1. In a large pan, heat sesame oil over medium heat. Add red chili flakes and toast for a few seconds.

2. Add ground chicken to the pan and cook until browned. Stir in ginger and garlic and cook for an additional 2 to 3 minutes.

3. Mix in tomato paste, soy sauce, and vegetablc broth. Let simmer to reduce by half.

4. In a small bowl, mix together cornstarch and water. Stir into the sauce and simmer on low heat for 2 minutes. The sauce will slightly thicken.

5. Gently stir in tofu and green onions. Cook for 5 minutes until the tofu has just warmed through.

Pork and apple skillet dinner

Ingredients

- 5 mL (1 tsp) vegetable oil

- 2 cloves garlic, minced

- 5 mL (1 tsp) dried thyme leaves

- 1 mL (¼ tsp) ground pepper

- 4 boneless pork loin chops (about 450 g/1 lb)

- 2 red skinned apples, cored and sliced

- 125 mL (½ cup) sodium-reduced chicken or vegetable broth

- 5 mL (1 tsp) Dijon mustard

- 2 mL (½ tsp) cornstarch

Directions

1. In a bowl, combine oil, garlic, thyme and pepper; add pork chops and rub mixture all over.

2. Heat a large non-stick skillet over medium-high heat and brown pork chops on both sides. Remove to plate and add apple slices to pan; cook, stirring for 2 minutes.

3. Whisk together broth, mustard and cornstarch; pour into skillet. Stir to coat apples. Return pork chops to skillet and cook, turning once, for about 3 minutes. Use a digital food thermometer to check that the pork has reached an internal temperature of 71 °C (160 °F).

BBQ chicken drumsticks

Ingredients

- 5 mL (1 tsp) vegetable oil

- 1 onion, chopped

- 2 cloves garlic, minced

- 15 mL (1 tbsp) chopped fresh thyme

- 10 mL (2 tsp) chili powder

- 1 mL (¼ tsp) ground pepper

- 500 mL (2 cups) passata (strained crushed tomatoes)

- 175 mL (¾ cup) chopped pitted Medjool dates

- 60 mL (¼ cup) cider vinegar

- 15 mL (1 tbsp) Worcestershire sauce

- 5 mL (1 tsp) hot pepper sauce

- 10 skinless chicken drumsticks (about 900 g)

Directions

1. In a saucepan, heat oil over medium heat and cook onion, garlic, thyme, chili powder

and pepper for 3 minutes or until softened. Stir in passata, dates, vinegar, Worcestershire and hot pepper sauce and bring to a simmer for 5 minutes. Remove from heat and let cool slightly. Scrape into blender and purée until smooth. Makes about 625 mL (2 ½ cups) of sauce.

2. Place drumsticks on greased grill over medium heat for 10 minutes. Turn and grill for 5 minutes more. Start brushing with about 250 mL (1 cup) of sauce, turning often and basting for about 10 more minutes. Use a digital food thermometer to check that chicken has reached an internal temperature of 74°C (165°F).

3. Serve with some of the remaining sauce, if desired.

Chicken fried rice

Ingredients

- 30 mL (2 tbsp.) vegetable oil, divided

- 2 eggs, lightly beaten

- 375 mL (1 ½ cups) chopped (into ½-inch pieces) cooked chicken breast

- 4 garlic cloves, minced

- 20 mL (1 ½ tbsp) minced fresh ginger

- 1 onion, finely diced

- 3 pieces baby bok choy, root trimmed and leaves finely chopped

- 1 L (4 cups) cooked brown rice, chilled or at room temperature

- 40 mL (2 ½ tbsp) lower sodium soy sauce

- 5 mL (1 tsp) sesame oil

- 4 scallions, thinly sliced

Directions

1. In a large wok or high-sided sauté pan, heat 15 mL (1 tbsp) of vegetable oil over medium-high heat. Pour eggs into the wok and scramble for about 1 minute or until just cooked through. Transfer to a plate and set aside.

2. Add chicken to the wok and heat for about 4 minutes, stirring occasionally. Transfer chicken to the plate with eggs.

3. Heat the remaining 15 mL (1 tbsp) of oil in the wok. Add garlic and ginger and cook for 1 minute over high heat. Add onion and

bok choy and sauté for about 3 minutes or until golden. Add rice, soy sauce, and sesame oil. Mix well to break up rice and spread seasoning around.

4. Add cooked eggs, chicken and 30 mL (2 tbsp) of the scallions. Stir-fry for about 2 minutes or until rice is hot.

5. Transfer to a serving bowl and sprinkle with remaining scallions.

Hot and sweet curried squash

Ingredients

- 15 mL (1 tbsp) canola oil

- 1 onion, minced

- 1 mL (¼ tsp) ground cumin

- 15 mL (1 tbsp) curry powder

- 2 garlic cloves, minced

- 1 L (4 cups) lower sodium vegetable broth, divided

- 1 medium butternut squash, peeled and diced (about 900 g/2 lb)

- 1 can (540 mL/19 oz) no salt added chickpeas, drained and rinsed

- 1 can (540 mL/19 oz) no salt added diced tomatoes, with juice

- 250 mL (1 cup) frozen mango, thawed and chopped

- Salt and pepper to taste

Directions

1. In a large pot, heat oil over medium heat. Add onion and cumin and cook for 3 minutes, stirring frequently.

2. Add curry powder and cook for 2 more minutes, stirring to keep from burning.

3. Add garlic and 500 mL (2 cups) of broth and bring to a simmer.

4. Add remaining broth, squash, chickpeas, and tomatoes to the pot. Bring back to a simmer and cook covered, for 25 minutes, stirring occasionally.

5. Add mango and cook for 5 minutes. Serve hot over brown rice.

Tofu rice bowl

Ingredients

Quick pickle:

- 1 carrot

- 3 radishes, thinly sliced

- 250 mL (1 cup) water

- 125 mL (½ cup) white vinegar

- 3 cloves garlic

- 2 mL (½ tsp) black pepper

- 15 mL (1 tbsp) salt

- 15 mL (1 tbsp) sugar

Tofu crumble:

- 375 mL (1 ½ cups) uncooked brown rice

- 15 mL (1 tbsp) sesame oil

- 10 mL (2 tsp) grated ginger

- 1 package (400 g/14 oz) firm tofu, crumbled

- 30 mL (2 tbsp) hoisin sauce

- 15 mL (1 tbsp) lime juice (about ½ lime)

- 30 mL (2 tbsp) lower sodium soy sauce

- 2 mL (½ tsp) dried basil

- 45 mL (3 tbsp) water

Sriracha dressing:

- 5 mL (1 tsp) sriracha

- 85 mL (⅓ cup) lower fat Greek yogurt

- 5 mL (1 tsp) lime juice

To assemble:

- ½ large cucumber, sliced

- ½ bell pepper, cut into thin strips

- ½ bunch cilantro (optional)

Directions

1. Prepare the quick pickle: Use a vegetable peeler to slice carrots into ribbons. Place into a small bowl or glass jar. Place radishes in a separate bowl or glass jar.

2. In a small pot, bring water, vinegar, garlic, pepper, salt and sugar to a boil. Pour

over carrots and radishes and let marinate for at least 20 minutes.

3. Cook rice per package instructions.

4. Prepare the tofu crumble: In a large pan, heat sesame oil and ginger over medium heat and cook for 1 minute. Add crumbled tofu and warm through while stirring.

5. Pour in hoisin sauce, 15 mL (1 tbsp) lime juice, soy sauce, and basil. Stir well and add water. Cook until half of the water evaporates. Remove from heat.

6. Prepare the sriracha dressing: Mix sriracha, yogurt, and 5 mL (1 tsp) lime juice together.

7. Serve tofu on rice. Top with cucumber, bell peppers, cilantro, pickled carrots, pickled radishes, and dressing.

Crunchy turkey fingers with oven fries

Ingredients

- 1 boneless skinless turkey breast (about 600 g)

- 15 mL (1 tbsp) Dijon or yellow mustard

- 5 mL (1 tsp) vegetable oil

- 500 mL (2 cups) bran flakes

- 30 mL (2 tbsp) grated Parmesan cheese

- 5 mL (1 tsp) Italian herb seasoning or dried oregano leaves

Oven Fries:

- 1 sweet potato, peeled and cut into strips

- 2 parsnips, peeled and cut into strips

- 5 mL (1 tsp) vegetable oil

- 2 mL (½ tsp) chili powder

Directions

1. Preheat the oven to 220 °C (425 °F).

2. Cut turkey breast into finger size strips and place in a bowl. Add mustard and oil and using your hands coat turkey fingers evenly.

3. Place bran flakes into a large resealable bag and crush to look like breadcrumbs. Add cheese and seasoning. Add turkey fingers to bag, one at a time, and shake to coat. Place coated turkey onto parchment paper lined

baking sheet. Repeat with all the turkey fingers; set aside.

4. Oven Fries: In a large bowl, combine sweet potato and parsnip strips. Add oil and chili powder and toss to coat evenly. On a second parchment paper lined baking sheet, spread fries in single layer onto sheet.

5. Place fries in bottom third of preheated oven for 15 minutes. Move fries to top third of oven and place turkey fingers on bottom third of oven for 15 minutes. Use a digital food thermometer to check that turkey has reached an internal temperature of 74°C (165°F).

Tomato and ricotta pasta

Ingredients

- 1 package (375 g) whole grain rotini or fusilli

- 10 mL (2 tsp) extra virgin olive oil

- 1 zucchini, grated

- 1 carrot, grated

- ½ red bell pepper, finely sliced

- 15 mL (1 tbsp) dried oregano

- 5 mL (1 tsp) dried basil

- 1 jar (700 mL) passata (strained crushed tomatoes)

- 125 mL (½ cup) water

- 45 mL (3 tbsp) chopped fresh parsley or basil

- 250 mL (1 cup) light ricotta cheese

- 30 mL (2 tbsp) grated Parmesan cheese (optional)

Directions

1. In a pot of boiling water, cook pasta for about 8 minutes or until tender but firm. Drain well and return pasta to pot; set aside.

2. Prepare the pasta sauce: Meanwhile, in a large and deep nonstick skillet, heat oil and cook zucchini, carrot, pepper, oregano and basil over medium heat for about 5 minutes or until starting to turn golden. Stir in

passata, water and parsley. Bring to a boil and simmer for 5 minutes.

3. Stir in ricotta, Parmesan cheese (optional), and pasta.

Black bean and corn salad

Ingredients

Salad:

- 1 can (540 mL/19 oz) no salt added black beans, rinsed and drained

- 1 can (540 mL/19 oz) no salt added corn kernels, rinsed and drained

- 2 tomatoes, chopped finely

- 1 red bell pepper, diced

- 60 mL (¼ cup) cilantro, chopped

- 190 mL (¾ cup) cooked chicken, diced

Dressing:

- 15 mL (1 tbsp) lime juice (about ½ lime)

- 15 mL (1 tbsp) olive oil

- 2 mL (½ tsp) ground cumin

- 2 mL (½ tsp) garlic powder

- Salt and pepper to taste

Directions

1. In a large salad bowl, combine black beans, corn, tomatoes, bell pepper, cilantro and cooked chicken.

2. In a small bowl, whisk dressing ingredients. Drizzle over top of salad and toss to coat.

Three sisters tacos

Ingredients

Squash:

- 1 medium butternut squash (about 1 kg/2 ¼ lb)

- 10 mL (2 tsp) olive oil

- 5 mL (1 tsp) chili powder

- 5 mL (1 tsp) dried oregano

Refried Beans:

- 15 mL (1 tbsp) olive oil

- 2 garlic cloves, peeled

- 1 ½ cans (1 ½ x 540 mL/19 oz) no salt added black beans, drained and rinsed

- 5 mL (1 tsp) ground cumin

- 30 mL (2 tbsp) lime juice (about 1 lime)

- 5 mL (1 tsp) chili powder

Tacos:

- 12 small whole grain corn tortillas

- 125 mL (½ cup) light feta cheese or queso fresco

Directions

1. Preheat the oven to 175 °C (350 °F). Peel squash, slice in half, and scoop out seeds. Chop squash into 1x3-inch sticks and place in a medium bowl.

2. Drizzle 10 mL (2 tsp) of olive oil over squash and season with chili powder and dried oregano. Toss to coat then transfer on parchment paper lined baking sheet and arrange squash in an even layer. Roast for 20 minutes or until nicely browned and tender inside. Remove from heat and let them cool.

3. In a high-sided skillet, heat 15 mL (1 tbsp) of olive oil over medium-high heat. Add the garlic cloves and cook for 4 to 5 minutes or until brown on both side, turning

once. In the skillet, mash garlic cloves with a fork.

4. Stir in black beans, ground cumin and chili powder and add 500 mL (2 cups) of water. Reduce to a simmer and cook for 10 minutes, stirring occasionally.

5. Mash bean mixture to the texture of a thick, chunky paste with a potato masher or a fork. Cook beans for 2 more minutes, stirring constantly. Remove from heat, add lime juice and stir to combine.

6. In a skillet over medium-high heat, warm tortillas. Transfer them into a clean kitchen towel to keep them warm. Spread a spoonful of the beans, 2 or 3 chunks of squash, and crumbled cheese. Season with salt to taste.

Smoked fish and white hominy corn soup

Ingredients

- 20 mL (1 ½ tbsp) sunflower oil

- 125 mL (½ cup) wild or commercial leeks, finely chopped

- 15 mL (1 tbsp) fresh sage, chopped

- 15 mL (1 tbsp) fresh mint, chopped

- 4 smoked fish fillets (about 200 g)

- 30 mL (2 tbsp) maple syrup, divided

- 1.5-2 L (6-8 cups) water

- 1 ½ cans (1 ½ x 540mL/19 oz) white hominy corn

Directions

1. In a large soup pot, heat oil over medium heat. Sauté leeks, sage, and mint for 2 minutes or until tender.

2. Add smoked fish, 15 mL (1 tbsp) maple syrup, and enough water to cover by about 7.5 cm (3 inches). Bring to a boil, then reduce heat to low. Simmer for 30 minutes.

3. Drain and rinse hominy and stir into soup. Season with 15 mL (1 tbsp) maple syrup.

Beef fajitas with lime sour cream

Ingredients

- 2 small beef grilling steaks, excess fat trimmed (about 400 g/12 oz)

- 10 mL (2 tsp) chili powder

- 2 mL (½ tsp) ground cumin

- 2 mL (½ tsp) black pepper

- 10 mL (2 tsp) vegetable oil, divided

- 1 onion, thinly sliced

- 2 red, orange or yellow bell peppers, thinly sliced

- 85 mL (⅓ cup) chopped fresh cilantro

- 6 small whole grain or corn tortillas

Lime Sour Cream:

- 60 mL (¼ cup) light sour cream

- 2 mL (½ tsp) grated lime zest

- 30 mL (2 tbsp) lime juice

Directions

1. Using a large knife, thinly slice steak crosswise into thin strips. Toss with chili powder, cumin and pepper.

2. In a non-stick skillet, heat half of the oil over medium high heat and brown beef. Remove to plate. Add remaining oil in same skillet and sauté onion, bell peppers and cilantro for 4 minutes or until tender crisp. Return beef to skillet and heat through.

3. For the lime sour cream, in a small bowl, stir together sour cream, lime zest and lime juice.

4. Divide beef-vegetable mixture among tortillas and top with lime sour cream.

SNACKS RECIPE SUGGESTIONS

Oat and pumpkin no-bake bites

Ingredients

• 750 mL (3 cups) rolled oats

• 250 mL (1 cup) pumpkin puree (not pumpkin pie filling)

• 250 mL (1 cup) natural almond or peanut butter or non-nut alternative

• 125 mL (½ cup) maple syrup

• 5 mL (1 tsp) cinnamon

• 7 mL (½ tbsp) vanilla

Directions

1. In a large bowl, combine all **ingredients** and mix well. If mixture is too dry, add more nut butter; if mixture is too wet, add more oats.

2. Using a tablespoon, scoop mixture in your hand and shape into 2.5 cm (1-inch) balls. Place on a baking sheet.

3. Cover and freeze for one hour before eating!

Peach, roasted chickpeas and halloumi cheese salad

Ingredients

- 30 mL (2 tbsp) olive oil, divided

- 1 can (540 mL/19 oz) lower sodium chickpeas, drained and rinsed

- 2 mL (½ tsp) paprika

- 5 mL (1 tsp) dried thyme

- 5 mL (1 tsp) garlic powder

- 3 peaches, sliced in wedges

- ½ package (100 g/3.5 oz) halloumi cheese, sliced

- 500 mL (2 cups) cherry tomatoes, halved

- 1 mL (¼ tsp) dried basil

- 15 mL (1 tbsp) lemon juice (about ½ lemon)

Directions

1. In a non-stick pan, add 15 mL (1 tbsp) of olive oil and toast chickpeas over medium-high heat for 10 minutes or until golden.

2. Pour into a large bowl and toss with paprika, thyme, and garlic powder.

3. Pre-heat a grill pan or BBQ to medium-high heat. Grill peaches and halloumi cheese for 3 minutes to warm through, until there are grill marks.

4. Dice the halloumi cheese into smaller pieces and add to the bowl with spiced chickpeas along with grilled peaches.

5. Stir in tomatoes, dried basil, and lemon juice. Coat with remaining 15 mL (1 tbsp) of olive oil.

Muhammara dip (red bell pepper and walnut)

Ingredients

- 2 red bell peppers

- 125 mL (½ cup) unsalted walnuts, divided

- 15 mL (1 tbsp) olive oil

- 1 clove garlic

- 2 mL (½ tsp) salt

- 1 mL (¼ tsp) paprika

- 2 mL (½ tsp) honey

- 30 mL (2 tbsp) breadcrumbs

Directions

1. Preheat the oven to 230 °C (450 °F) and line 2 baking sheets with aluminum foil.

2. Place red bell peppers on a baking sheet. Roast for 30 to 40 minutes or until peppers are soft and skins begin to blacken, checking from time to time. Let cool and remove stems and seeds.

3. Roast walnuts on a separate tray for 2 to 3 minutes.

4. Place half of walnuts in a zip top bag and let kids crush with a mallet. Reserve.

5. In a blender, place bell peppers, oil, uncrushed walnut, garlic, salt, paprika, and honey. Blend until smooth.

6. Empty into a bowl and stir in crushed walnuts and breadcrumbs.

Apple berry crisp

Ingredients

- 4 apples, cored and chopped

- 500 mL (2 cups) frozen or fresh blueberries

- 45 mL (3 tbsp) packed brown sugar

- 30 mL (2 tbsp) all purpose flour

- 5 mL (1 tsp) vanilla

Topping:

- 250 mL (1 cup) large flake oats

- 125 mL (½ cup) all purpose flour

- 85 mL (⅓ cup) wheat bran

- 30 mL (2 tbsp) packed brown sugar

- 2 mL (½ tsp) ground cinnamon

- 45 mL (3 tbsp) soft non-hydrogenated margarine, melted

Directions

1. Preheat the oven to 180 °C (350 °F).

2. In a large bowl, combine apples, blueberries, sugar, flour and vanilla and stir until well-coated. Spread into a 20 cm/8 in square baking dish; set aside.

3. Prepare the topping: In another bowl, combine oats, flour, wheat bran, sugar and cinnamon. Add melted margarine and using

a fork, toss to coat oat mixture. Sprinkle over top of fruit mixture.

4. Bake for about 50 minutes or until apples are tender and the top is golden. Let cool slightly before serving.

Cantaloupe and bocconcini cheese salad

Ingredients

- 30 mL (2 tbsp) lime juice (about 1 lime)

- 20 mL (1 ½ tbsp) olive oil

- 2 mL (½ tsp) salt

- 1 mL (¼ tsp) black pepper

- 30 mL (2 tbsp) chopped fresh mint

- 1 cantaloupe, diced small

- 125 mL (½ cup) chopped bocconcini cheese

- 250 mL (1 cup) cherry tomatoes, halved

- 60 mL (¼ cup) thinly sliced red onion

- 60 mL (¼ cup) unsalted almonds, toasted and roughly chopped

- 60 mL (¼ cup) unsalted pumpkin seeds

Directions

1. In a large bowl, whisk together lime juice, olive oil, salt, pepper, and mint.

2. Add cantaloupe, bocconcini, tomatoes, and onion.

3. Toss well and top with almonds and pumpkin seeds when ready to serve.

Savoury pear and cheese scones

Ingredients

- 375 mL (1 ½ cups) whole wheat flour

- 125 mL (½ cup) oat bran

- 10 mL (2 tsp) baking powder

- 10 mL (2 tsp) packed brown sugar

- 1 mL (¼ tsp) ground nutmeg

- 30 mL (2 tbsp) soft non-hydrogenated margarine

- 165 mL (⅔ cup) 0% plain Greek yogurt

- 1 ripe pear, cored and diced

- 85 mL (⅓ cup) shredded light old Cheddar or crumbled blue cheese

Directions

1. Preheat the oven to 200 °C (400 °F) and line a baking sheet with parchment paper.

2. In a large bowl, combine flour, oat bran, baking powder, sugar and nutmeg. Using your fingers or a pastry blender, rub margarine into flour mixture until it looks crumbly. Using a fork, stir in yogurt to make a ragged dough. Add pear and cheese and knead gently to make a soft dough.

3. Place dough on a floured surface and pat into a 20 cm (8 inch) circle about 2 cm (¾ inch) thick and cut into 8 wedges. Separate wedges and place on baking sheet.

4. Bake for about 15 minutes or until golden.

Cornbread

Ingredients

• 30 mL (2 tbsp) light sour cream

• 310 mL (1 ¼ cups) lower fat milk or unsweetened fortified plant-based beverage

• 60 mL (¼ cup) sunflower oil

• 2 eggs

• 335 mL (1 ⅓ cups) whole wheat flour

• 165 mL (⅔ cup) medium grind cornmeal

• 165 mL (⅔ cup) granulated sugar

- 15 mL (1 tbsp) baking powder

- 2 mL (½ tsp) salt

Directions

1. Preheat the oven to 175°C (350°F). Mist a 20x20 cm (8x8-inch) pan with non-stick spray or line with parchment paper.

2. In a large bowl, whisk sour cream, milk, oil, and eggs together.

3. In a separate bowl, whisk together flour, cornmeal, sugar, baking powder, and salt. Add to the large bowl and stir until combined.

4. Transfer batter to the pan and bake for 35 to 45 minutes, or until fluffy and slightly golden around the edges. A toothpick

inserted into the centre should come out clean or with a few moist crumbs.

5. Cool in the pan for about 20 minutes. Cut into 16 square pieces and serve.

Curried chickpea salad

Ingredients

• 1 can (540 mL/19 oz) lower sodium chickpeas, drained and rinsed

• 45 mL (3 tbsp) lower fat yogurt

• 60 mL (¼ cup) diced celery

• ¼ red onion, diced

• 60 mL (¼ cup) raisins

- 1 tomato, diced

- 2 mL (½ tsp) curry powder

- 15 mL (1 tbsp) apricot jam (optional)

- 7 mL (½ tbsp) lemon juice (about ½ lemon)

- 1 mL (¼ tsp) black pepper

- Pinch of salt

Directions

1. In a large bowl, place chickpeas and roughly mash with a fork or potato masher.

2. Add all remaining **ingredients** and toss to combine.

3. Cover and marinate in the refrigerator for 10 to 15 minutes.

Cauliflower and bean dip

Ingredients

- 1 head cauliflower, cut into small florets

- 30 mL (2 tbsp) olive oil, divided

- 1 can (540 mL/19 oz) no salt added white kidney beans, drained and rinsed

- 2 mL (½ tsp) garlic powder

- 2 mL (½ tsp) paprika

- 2 mL (½ tsp) lemon juice (about ¼ lemon)

- 125 mL (½ cup) water

- Salt and pepper to taste

Directions

1. Preheat the oven to 190 °C (375 °F).

2. In a large bowl, toss cauliflower with 15 mL (1 tbsp) oil until well-coated.

3. Spread cauliflower on a non-stick baking sheet and roast for 45 minutes or until soft, turning over halfway to keep from burning. Let cool.

4. In a blender or food processor, blend cauliflower, beans, garlic powder, paprika, lemon juice, water, remaining olive oil, and salt. Mix until smooth.

5. Transfer dip to a serving bowl.

Zesty bean dip and baked chips

Ingredients

- 6 small whole grain flour or corn tortillas

- 4 mL (¾ tsp) chili powder

- 1 can (540 mL/19 oz) black beans, drained and rinsed

- 125 mL (½ cup) medium or hot salsa

- 1 mL (¼ tsp) grated lime zest

- 30 mL (2 tbsp) lime juice (about 1 lime)

- 1 small shallot, minced

- 2 mL (½ tsp) ground cumin

- Pinch ground pepper

- 45 mL (3 tbsp) chopped fresh cilantro

- 30 mL (2 tbsp) chopped fresh basil (optional)

Directions

1. Preheat the oven to 200 °C (400 °F).

2. Cut each tortilla into 8 wedges and place in a resealable plastic bag. Spray tortillas with cooking spray and sprinkle with chili powder; seal and shake bag to coat tortilla wedges. Place on large baking sheet and bake in preheated oven for about 8 minutes or until golden and crisp. Let cool completely before using.

3. In a food processor, purée beans, salsa, lime zest, lime juice, shallot, cumin and pepper until smooth. Scrape into bowl and stir in cilantro and basil, if using.

4. Serve with tortilla chips.

Creamy hummus

Ingredients

• 1 can (540 mL/19 oz) sodium-reduced chickpeas, drained and rinsed

• 60 mL (¼ cup) tahini (sesame seed paste)

• 5 mL (1 tsp) ground cumin

• 60 mL (¼ cup) sodium-reduced vegetable broth

• 2 mL (½ tsp) grated lemon zest

• 15 mL (1 tbsp) lemon juice (about ½ lemon)

- 30 mL (2 tbsp) water (or more as desired)

- 1 clove garlic, minced

Directions

1. In a food processor, combine chickpeas, tahini and cumin. Pulse until coarse.

2. Add broth, lemon zest, lemon juice, and water. Pulse until smooth; add more water as necessary for a creamy texture. Stir in garlic.

Lentil nuggets

Ingredients

- 1 can (540 mL/19 oz) lentils, drained and rinsed

- 60 mL (¼ cup) rolled oats

- 30 mL (2 tbsp) lemon juice (about 1 lemon)

- 10 mL (2 tsp) dried basil

- 10 mL (2 tsp) cumin

- 5 mL (1 tsp) garlic powder

- 15 mL (1 tbsp) olive oil

Directions

1. In a blender or food processor, place all **ingredients** (except for olive oil) and blend until smooth.

2. Form mini patties with your hands by rolling about 15 mL (1 tbsp) of the mixture and then molding into the shape of little

disks (or any other shape you like). Place patties on a plate.

3. In a large skillet, heat olive oil over medium-high heat. Gently transfer the nuggets to the skillet and pan-fry for about 2 to 3 minutes per side or until golden brown on both sides. Remove from skillet and allow to cool.

Carrot potato pancakes

Ingredients

- 4 eggs

- 500 mL (2 cups) finely grated carrot

- 500 mL (2 cups) finely grated potato

- 15 mL (1 tbsp) finely grated onion

- 30 mL (2 tbsp) whole wheat flour

- 2 mL (½ tsp) baking powder

Directions

1. Beat eggs in a large bowl. Stir in carrot, potato, onion, flour, and baking powder. Mix well.

2. Spray griddle or non-stick skillet lightly with cooking spray. Heat over medium heat. Using 125 mL (½ cup) measuring cup, pour batter onto hot griddle. Cook for about 2 minutes or until light golden brown. Flip over and cook for another minute or until light golden brown. Repeat with remaining batter.

Tofu and berry sheet tart

Ingredients

- 375 mL (1 ½ cups) frozen mixed berries

- 30 mL (2 tbsp) cornstarch

- 1 package (300 g/10.5 oz) soft tofu

- 15 mL (1 tbsp) honey

- 5 mL (1 tsp) vanilla extract

- 1 sheet (225 g/8 oz) puff pastry, thawed

- 125 mL (½ cup) unsalted pumpkin seeds

Directions

1. Preheat the oven to 190 °C (375 °F) and line a baking sheet with parchment paper.

2. in a small bowl, mix berries and cornstarch together. Set aside.

3. Drain excess liquid from the tofu. In a separate bowl, mash until smooth and stir in honey and vanilla extract.

4. Roll out the puff pastry into roughly a 23x30 cm (9x12 inch) rectangle. Place onto the baking sheet. Spread tofu on top, making sure to leave a 2.5 cm (1 inch) border. Spoon mixed berries onto tofu.

5. Bake for 25 to 30 minutes, until the edges are golden brown and fruits bubble.

6. Remove from the oven and top with pumpkin seeds or your family's favorite nuts or seeds.

Puff bars

Ingredients

- 1 L (4 cups) wheat, rice, or Kamut puffs

- 45 mL (3 tbsp) chia seeds

- 60 mL (¼ cup) unsalted pumpkin seeds

- 45 mL (3 tbsp) cacao nibs or mini chocolate chips

- 85 mL (⅓ cup) natural peanut or almond butter or non-nut alternative

- 85 mL (⅓ cup) honey

Directions

1. Line a 20x20 cm (8x8 inch) square pan with parchment paper and set aside.

2. In a large bowl, mix together puffs, chia seeds, pumpkin seeds, and cacao nibs.

3. In a microwave safe bowl, add peanut butter and honey. Microwave in 20-second intervals stirring in between each interval until mixture is smooth and pourable.

4. Pour warm peanut butter mixture over puff mixture and mix well.

5. Press mixture into the pan and place in the freezer for 30 minutes.

6. Cut into 12 portions.

Tuna and tomato salad

Ingredients

- 1 L (2 pints) grape tomatoes, halved lengthwise

- 2 stalks celery, thinly sliced

- 2 cans (each 120 g drained weight) light flaked tuna in water, drained

- 250 mL (1 cup) chopped cucumber

Salad dressing:

- 45 mL (3 tbsp) red wine vinegar

- 10 mL (2 tsp) extra virgin olive oil

- 1 clove garlic, minced

- Pinch hot pepper flakes

- 85 mL (⅓ cup) chopped fresh basil

- 30 mL (2 tbsp) chopped fresh oregano

Directions

1. In a large bowl, combine tomatoes, celery, tuna and cucumber.

2. Prepare the salad dressing: In a small bowl, whisk together vinegar, oil, garlic and hot pepper flakes. Pour over tomato mixture along with basil and oregano and toss to coat well.

Fruit and yogurt granola parfaits

Ingredients

- 250 mL (1 cup) steel cut oats

- 250 mL (1 cup) large flake oats

- 165 mL (⅔ cup) slivered almonds

- 85 mL (⅓ cup) wheat germ

- 60 mL (¼ cup) flaxseed meal

- 45 mL (3 tbsp) pure maple syrup

- 15 mL (1 tbsp) vanilla

- 30 mL (2 tbsp) vegetable oil

- 1 L (4 cups) 0% plain Greek yogurt

- 750 mL (3 cups) fresh or frozen berries, such as raspberries, blueberries or blackberries

Directions

1. Preheat the oven to 180 °C (350 °F).

2. On a large baking sheet, spread steel-cut oats, large flake oats, almonds, wheat germ and flaxseed meal in single layer. Bake in preheated oven, stirring a couple of times, for about 15 minutes or until light golden. Scrape into a bowl.

3. In a small bowl, whisk together maple syrup, vanilla and oil. Pour over oat mixture and stir to coat evenly. Spread mixture onto baking sheet and return to oven for about 15 minutes or until golden brown, stirring at least twice. Let cool completely.

4. When ready to serve, divide half the granola among 10 small glasses or parfait dishes. Divide yogurt among glasses and sprinkle with some fruit. Top with remaining granola and fruit and enjoy. Alternatively, cover and refrigerate for up to a day.

Fruit skewers with maple yogurt dip

Ingredients

Skewers:

• 8 strawberries, halved

• 2 peaches, sliced into 8 wedges each

• 2 bananas, peeled and each cut into 8 pieces

Yogurt dip:

- 250 mL (1 cup) 0% plain Greek yogurt

- 15 mL (1 tbsp) pure maple syrup

- 2 mL (½ tsp) ground cinnamon

Directions

1. Pierce fruit onto small skewers, alternating fruit.

2. In a bowl, whisk together yogurt, maple syrup and cinnamon. Serve with fruit skewers.

Apple sandwiches

Ingredients

- 60 (¼ cup) natural almond or peanut butter or non-nut alternative

- 85 mL (⅓ cup) 0% plain Greek yogurt

- Sprinkle of cinnamon

- 2 apples, cored and thinly sliced horizontally

- Optional toppings: sliced almonds, dried fruit, unsweetened shredded coconut, seeds

Directions

1. In a small bowl, combine nut or non-nut butter with Greek yogurt and cinnamon. Stir until combined.

2. On a clean cutting board, lay apple slices and spread about 10 mL (2 tsp) of yogurt/nut butter mix on each. Add toppings of choice!

Crispy chickpeas

Ingredients

- 1 can (540 mL/19 oz) no salt added chickpeas, drained and rinsed

- 15 mL (1 tbsp) vegetable oil

- 2 mL (½ tsp) dried thyme

- 2 mL (½ tsp) ground pepper

Directions

1. Preheat the oven to 180°C (350°F).

2. Spread chickpeas onto one end of a clean towel. Fold the other side of the towel over chickpeas and gently roll them in between the two ends to dry. As they dry, some skins will come off. Remove as many skins as possible and continue to pat dry. The drier they are, the more they will crisp up when baking.

3. Toss chickpeas in oil and spread evenly on a rimmed baking sheet.

4. Bake for 25 minutes. Remove from the oven, add thyme and ground pepper and stir to ensure they are well coated and so they brown evenly.

5. Return to the oven and bake for another 15 to 20 minutes, or until golden brown and crispy.

6. Remove the pan from the oven and let them cool; they will continue to crisp up as they cool. These are best eaten the same day to maintain their crispiness.

DESSERTS RECIPE SUGGESTIONS

Tasty Galaxy Stuffed Cookies

Ingredients

for 12 servings

• 1 Tasty Galaxy Stuffed Cookies Dessert Kit

• 4 tablespoons water, divided

• 4 tablespoons butter, softened, divided

Preparation

1. Preheat the oven to 375°F.

2. Beat Blue Cookie Mix, 2 tablespoons butter, and 2 tablespoons water in a medium mixing bowl with a hand mixer until dough forms. Repeat with Purple Cookie Mix and remaining 2 tablespoons of butter and water.

3. Freeze both doughs for 20 minutes.

4. Roll each batch of chilled dough into a 12-inch log; place, side by side, on a floured work surface, then tightly twist logs together. Roll to form rope.

5. Break off 6 rectangles of the white chocolate bar, then break each small rectangle in half. Reserve the remaining white chocolate bar for later use.

6. Form dough into 12 balls, using about 1 tablespoon of dough for each ball; flatten

each ball into 2-inch round. Place 1 square of white chocolate on the center of each round. Mold dough around the chocolate to completely enclose chocolate; place on a parchment-covered baking sheet.

7. Bake 12–13 minutes or until puffed in the centers and set around the edges. Cool for 5 minutes before transferring cookies to a cooling rack.

8. Microwave reserved white chocolate bar in microwaveable bowl on high for 1 minute or until completely melted, stirring after 30 seconds. Drizzle the chocolate over warm cookies; top with pink sprinkles.

9. Enjoy!

Caramel Apple Crumble

Ingredients

for 8 servings

- 8 granny smith apples, peeled, cored, and cut into 1-inch (2.5 cm) pieces

- 2 tablespoons all-purpose flour

BAILEYS CARAMEL SAUCE

- 2 sticks unsalted butter

- 2 cups brown sugar (220 g), lightly packed

- 1 cup Baileys Apple Pie (240 mL)

- 1 teaspoon vanilla extract

- 1 ½ tablespoons ground cinnamon

- 1 teaspoon kosher salt

CRUMBLE TOPPING

- 2 cups oats(160 g)

- 2 cups all purpose flour(250 g)

- ½ cup brown sugar(105 g), packed

- 2 teaspoons ground cinnamon

- 1 teaspoon baking powder

- 1 teaspoon kosher salt

- 2 sticks unsalted butter, melted

FOR SERVING

- 8 scoops vanilla ice cream

- 1 cup Baileys Apple Pie(240 mL)

Preparation

1. Preheat the oven to 350°F (180°C).

2. Add the apples to a large bowl and sprinkle with the flour. Toss to coat, then set aside.

3. Make the Baileys caramel sauce: Melt the butter in a large saucepan over medium heat. Add the brown sugar and whisk continuously for 1 minute, until the sugar starts to dissolve.

4. Add the Baileys Apple Pie and continue to whisk for 3–5 minutes, or until the caramel is smooth and starting to thicken. Whisk in the vanilla, cinnamon, and salt until incorporated.

5. Remove the pot from the heat and pour the caramel into the bowl with the apples, stirring to coat evenly.

6. Make the crumble topping: Add the oats, flour, brown sugar, cinnamon, baking powder and salt to a large bowl and stir to combine. Add the melted butter and mix until incorporated, with the consistency of wet sand.

7. To assemble, spread the caramel-coated apples in an even layer in a 9x13-inch (22 x 33 cm) baking dish. Sprinkle the crumble topping evenly over the top.

8. Bake the crumble for about 45 minutes or until the topping is golden brown and the juices are bubbling. Remove from the oven and let cool for 10–15 minutes.

9. Serve the crumble warm with vanilla ice cream and a drizzle of Baileys Apple Pie.

10. Enjoy!

Chocolate Oat Cookies

Ingredients

for 20 servings

- ¾ cup butter(170 g), melted

- 1 cup brown sugar(200 g)

- 1 egg

- 1 teaspoon vanilla extract

- 1 ½ cups kodiak cake mix(185 g)

- 1 cup oats(75 g)

- 1 tablespoon nutella

Preparation

1. Preheat the oven to 350°F.

2. Mix the sugar, cake mix, and oats. Add the eggs, vanilla, and butter to a separate bowl and cream together.

3. Add wet ingredient mixture to dry and mix well. Then, add Nutella, mix, and form into a dough.

4. Shape the dough into balls and arrange on a greased cookie sheet.

5. Bake for 12 minutes. Once golden, cool on a wire rack for 5 minutes.

6. Serve warm.

Sweet Fresh Corn Tamales

Ingredients

for 12 Tamales

- 12 Whole ears of corn

- 14 oz sweetened condensed milk

- ½ cup cane sugar

- 3 tablespoons ground cinnamon

- 1 teaspoon kosher salt

- ⅓ cup masa

Preparation

1. Remove the husks and silk from the corn, reserving the tender green leaves for wrapping.

2. Using a large, sharp knife, remove the kernels from the cob and place into a high powered blender. Blend the kernels until smooth and then pass the corn puree through a fine-mesh strainer set over a bowl to let the excess liquid drain.

3. Place the strained corn puree in a clean bowl and stir together with the sweetened condensed milk, cane sugar and cinnamon. Slowly drizzle in the masa until a thick batter forms.

4. Place a bamboo steamer over a pot of boiling water.

5. Place a corn husk on a flat surface with the pointed end away from you. Spoon about ½ cup of the corn puree into the middle. Snugly fold over the two long flaps like a business letter, then fold over a few

inches of the pointed end of the husk, creating a little bit of tension so that the tamales don't flatten while steaming. Repeat with the remaining filling and husks.

6. Carefully lay the tamales in the steamer in a single layer, working in batches if necessary. Cover the steamer basket and cook the tamales until they are slightly firm, about 15 minutes.

7. Enjoy!

Gingerbread Donuts

Ingredients

for 20 donuts

- 3 cups all purpose flour(375 g), plus more for dusting

- 1 teaspoon baking powder

- ½ teaspoon baking soda

- ¼ teaspoon kosher salt

- ¼ cup granulated sugar(25 g)

- ½ cup brown sugar(100 g)

- 2 teaspoons McCormick® ground ginger

- 1 ½ teaspoons McCormick® Ground Cinnamon

- ¼ teaspoon McCormick® Ground Cloves

- ¼ teaspoon McCormick® Ground Nutmeg

- 2 large eggs

- 1 stick unsalted butter, melted

- ⅓ cup molasses(80 mL)

- 2 teaspoons McCormick® vanilla extract

- ⅓ cup sour cream(80 mL)

- ½ cup whole milk(120 mL)

- vegetable oil, for frying

MCCORMICK® GINGER-CINNAMON BROWN SUGAR DUST

- ½ cup granulated sugar(100 g)

- ½ cup packed brown sugar(100 g)

- 2 teaspoons McCormick® ground ginger

- 3 teaspoons McCormick® Ground Cinnamon

SPECIAL EQUIPMENT

- 3-inch round cutter

- 1¼-inch round cutter

Preparation

1. In a large bowl and using a hand mixer, combine the flour, baking powder, baking soda, salt, granulated sugar, brown sugar, McCormick® Ground Ginger, McCormick® Ground Cinnamon, McCormick® Ground Cloves, and McCormick® Ground Nutmeg. Mix with a spatula until completely combined.

2. In a medium bowl or large liquid measuring cup, whisk together the eggs, melted butter, molasses, vanilla, sour cream, and milk.

3. Add the wet **ingredients** to the dry **ingredients** and mix on medium speed until fully combined and the batter is smooth and thick, about 3 minutes.

4. Turn the batter out onto a generously floured surface and dust more flour over the top and sides. Roll out to a 10x12-inch rectangle, about ¾ inch thick. Dip a 3-inch round cutter in flour, then cut out as many rounds of dough as possible, dipping the cutter in flour between each cut. Make sure the donuts are not sticking to the surface. Use a 1¼-inch round cutter to cut out the center of each donut. Reroll any scraps and cut out more donuts.

5. Make the McCormick® ginger-cinnamon brown sugar dust: In a medium bowl, whisk together the granulated sugar, brown sugar,

McCormick® Ground Ginger, and McCormick® Ground Cinnamon.

6. Fill a medium pot halfway with vegetable oil and heat over medium heat until the temperature reaches 350°F (180°C). Line a baking sheet with paper towels or a wire rack.

7. Working in batches of 4–5 at a time, fry the donuts in the hot oil until golden brown, 1–2 minutes per side. Use a spider or slotted spoon to transfer the donuts to the prepared baking sheet and let cool for 2 minutes. Toss 1–2 donuts at a time in the McCormick® ginger-cinnamon brown sugar dust to coat completely.

8. Serve warm or at room temperature.

9. Enjoy!

Cardamom Pistachio Sugar Cookies

Ingredients

for 48 servings

• 2 ¼ cups all purpose flour(280 g), plus more for dusting

• 1 teaspoon ground cardamom

• ½ teaspoon fine sea salt

• ¾ cup granulated sugar(150 g)

• ½ cup shelled pistachios(65 g), plus ¼ cup (30 g), very finely chopped

• 2 sticks unsalted butter, room temperature

• 1 large egg

- 1 teaspoon vanilla extract

- 2 ¾ cups powdered sugar(300 g)

- ¼ cup whole milk(60 mL)

- dried rose petal, for garnish - optional

Preparation

1. In a medium bowl, combine the flour, cardamom, and salt.

2. In a food processor, combine the granulated sugar and ½ cup (65 g) pistachios. Process until finely ground. Transfer to a stand mixer fitted with the paddle attachment.

3. Add the butter to the stand mixer bowl and beat on medium speed until smooth, 1 minute. Scrape down the sides of the bowl,

then add the egg and vanilla and beat until almost combined. Add the flour mixture and continue to mix on medium-low speed just until the dough comes together. Divide the dough into 2 portions and shape into discs. Wrap in plastic wrap and chill in the refrigerator for 1 hour.

4. Line 2 baking sheets with parchment paper.

5. Working with 1 portion at a time, roll out the dough on a lightly floured surface to ⅛ inch thick. Using a 2 ⅝-inch (6-cm) scalloped-edge cutter, cut out cookies, then transfer to the prepared baking sheets, spacing 1 inch apart. Re-roll the scraps to cut out more cookies. Chill in the refrigerator for 20 minutes.

6. Arrange the oven racks in the top and bottom third positions. Preheat to 350°F (180°C).

7. Bake the cookies, rotating the baking sheets 180° and swapping top to bottom halfway through, until the cookies have set, 12–14 minutes. Let cool on baking sheets for 5 minutes, then transfer to a wire rack to cool completely, about 20 minutes.

8. Combine the powdered sugar and milk in a small bowl and stir until smooth; the icing will be thick.

9. Using an offset spatula, spread the icing evenly over cookies, all the way to the edges. Return to the rack and immediately sprinkle the finely crushed pistachios and rose petals, if using, on top. Let sit until dry to the touch, 20 more minutes.

10. Enjoy!

Lemon-Lime Soda Cake As Made By Stefani

Ingredients

for 10 servings

CAKE

• nonstick cooking spray, for greasing

• 3 sticks unsalted butter, room temperature

• 2 ½ cups granulated sugar(500 g)

• 5 large eggs, room temperature

• 1 teaspoon vanilla extract

- 1 teaspoon lemon zest

- 2 tablespoons lemon

- 3 cups all purpose flour(375 g), spooned and leveled

- ½ teaspoon kosher salt

- ¾ cup lemon lime soda(180 mL), room temperature

GLAZE

- 1 ½ cups powdered sugar(165 g)

- 1 tablespoon lemon juice

- 1 teaspoon lime juice

- 1 tablespoon lemon lime soda

- ¼ teaspoon lime zest

- ¼ teaspoon lemon zest

Preparation

1. Preheat the oven to 325°F (160°C). Grease a 10–12 cup Bundt pan or tube pan (without a removable bottom).

2. In the bowl of a stand mixer fitted with a paddle attachment (or in a large bowl with an electric hand mixer), beat the butter on low speed for 2 minutes. Add the sugar and cream on high speed for about 5 minutes, until pale yellow, light, and fluffy.

3. Add the eggs, 1 at a time, and beat on low speed between each addition until just incorporated, scraping down the sides of the bowl as needed. Do not overmix. Add the vanilla, lemon zest, and lemon juice and mix for about 30 seconds, until combined. The

mixture will look a little curdled, but will smooth out once the flour is added.

4. Gradually add the flour and salt and mix until just combined. Using a rubber spatula, fold in the lemon-lime soda.

5. Pour the batter into the prepared pan and smooth the top. Bake for 60–75 minutes, until a toothpick inserted into the center of the cake comes out clean or with a few moist crumbs attached. Remove the cake from the oven and let cool in the pan for about 10 minutes, then invert onto a wire rack and let cool completely, about 1 hour.

6. Make the glaze: In a medium bowl, whisk together the powdered sugar, lemon juice, lime juice, and lemon-lime soda until completely smooth. Whisk in the lime and lemon zests.

7. Drizzle the glaze over the cake and let set for 5–10 minutes before serving.

8. Slice and serve.

9. Enjoy!

Red Velvet Shortbread Cookies

Ingredients

for 24 cookies

COOKIES

- 2 sticks unsalted butter, softened

- ¾ cup all purpose flour(95 g), plus more for dusting

- 1 box red velvet cake mix

- 3 tablespoons water

DECORATING

- 5 oz vanilla candy melts(140 g)

- white sanding sugar

- red sprinkle

- Red and green sprinkle

- white sprinkle

SPECIAL TOOLS

- Assorted 4-inch cookie cutter

Preparation

1. In a large bowl, use an electric mixer on medium speed to cream the butter until smooth, about 1 minute. Add the flour and mix until combined, about 30 seconds. Add the cake mix and water and continue mixing until smooth, about 1 minute more. Transfer the dough to a sheet of plastic wrap and flatten into a disc. Wrap tightly, then refrigerate until slightly firmed, about 30 minutes.

2. Preheat the oven to 350°F (180°C). Line 2 baking sheets with parchment paper.

3. Divide the dough in half. Working with one portion at a time (wrap the other in the plastic and refrigerate until ready to use), roll out on a lightly floured surface to ½ inch thick. Cut out shapes using the cookie

cutters. Use an offset spatula to gently lift the cookies and transfer to the prepared baking sheets, spacing 1 inch apart. Gather and re-roll the scraps until all of the dough is used.

4. Bake the cookies until they have puffed and the edges begin to crisp, 8–10 minutes. Remove from the oven and let cool for 5 minutes, then transfer to a wire rack to cool completely, about 30 minutes.

5. When ready to decorate, place the candy melts in a microwave-safe bowl and microwave in 30-second intervals, stirring between, until melted completely.

6. Line a baking sheet with parchment paper.

7. Dip the cookies in the candy melts, then place on the prepared baking sheet. Alternatively, transfer the candy melts to a small piping bag and cut the tip, then drizzle over the cookies. Garnish with the red, green, and white sprinkles. Let sit until the candy hardens, about 10 minutes.

8. Enjoy!

Lucky Charms Cereal Milk Cupcakes

Ingredients

for 12 cupcakes

CEREAL MILK

- 1 cup Lucky Charms™ Cereal(125 g)

- 1 ½ cups whole milk(360 mL)

CUPCAKES

- 1 ¾ cups cake flour(215 g)

- 2 teaspoons baking powder

- ¼ teaspoon kosher salt

- 1 stick unsalted butter, room temperature

- 1 cup granulated sugar(200 g)

- 2 large eggs, room temperature

- ⅓ cup sour cream(80 g), room temperature

- 2 ½ teaspoons vanilla extract

CEREAL MILK BUTTERCREAM

- ¼ cup all purpose flour(30 g)

- ¼ cup granulated sugar(50 g), plus 3 tablespoons

- 1 pinch kosher salt

- 1 ½ sticks unsalted butter, room temperature

- 1 teaspoon vanilla extract

TOPPINGS

- ½ cup Lucky Charms™ Marshmallows(30 g)

- 2 sheets edible gold leaf

Preparation

1. Make the cereal milk: Separate the marshmallows and cereal from the Lucky

Charms™ and set the marshmallows aside for assembling the cupcakes.

2. Add the cereal and milk to a large liquid measuring cup. Let the cereal soak for 20 minutes, stirring occasionally. Drain the cereal milk through a fine-mesh sieve into a clean liquid measuring cup. Discard the cereal and set the cereal milk aside.

3. Make the cupcakes: Preheat the oven to 350°F (180°C). Line a 12-cup muffin tin with paper liners.

4. In a medium bowl, whisk together the flour, baking powder, and salt.

5. In the bowl of a stand mixer fitted with the paddle attachment, beat the butter and sugar together on medium speed for about 3 minutes, or until light and fluffy.

6. Add the eggs, 1 at a time, beating between each addition until incorporated. Add the sour cream and vanilla, and beat until combined.

7. With the mixer running on low speed, alternate additions of the flour mixture and ¾ cup of the cereal milk until incorporated. Do not overmix.

8. Fill each cupcake liner with the batter to about ⅔ of the way full. Bake for 18–20 minutes, or until the tops of the cupcakes feel springy to the touch. Remove from the oven and let cool completely.

9. While the cupcakes are cooling, make the buttercream: Add the flour and remaining ¾ cup cereal milk to a small saucepan and whisk until all of the flour is incorporated. Place the saucepan over medium heat.

Cook, whisking continuously, for about 2 minutes, or until thickened. Immediately remove the pot from the heat and add the sugar and salt. Stir until the sugar has completely dissolved; the mixture will thin out after the sugar is added.

10. Transfer the mixture into a shallow dish and cover with plastic wrap, pressing directly against the surface to prevent a skin from forming. Transfer to the refrigerator for about 1 hour, until cool, but not fully chilled.

11. Once the flour mixture has cooled, beat the butter in the bowl of a stand mixer fitted with the whisk attachment until light and fluffy, about 3 minutes. Slowly add the flour mixture, 1 spoonful at a time, until completely incorporated. Add the vanilla, then increase the mixer speed to medium-

high and whip until the frosting is light and fluffy. (It should hold its shape on the whisk.) If the frosting is too runny, chill the bowl for 30 minutes before whipping again. If it is too thick and chunky, let sit at room temperature for 30 minutes before whipping again. Transfer the frosting to a piping bag fitted with a large open star tip.

12. Assemble the cupcakes: Cut out the center of each cupcake and fill each with 5–6 Lucky Charms™ Marshmallows. Pipe the buttercream in a swirl on top of each cupcake. Crush some of the remaining marshmallows between your fingertips and sprinkle on top of the cupcakes. Use a small, food-safe brush to apply small bits of gold leaf to the tops of the cupcakes, then place a whole marshmallow atop each cupcake.

13. Serve the cupcakes at room temperature. Leftover cupcakes will keep in an airtight container at room temperature for up to 3 days.

14. Enjoy!

Glutinous Rice Balls (Tang Yuan)

Ingredients

for 20 balls

FILLINGS

- ¼ cup black sesame seeds(35 g)

- ¼ cup unsalted peanuts(30 g)

- 4 tablespoons granulated sugar, divided

- 2 tablespoons unsalted butter, room temperature

BROWN SUGAR GINGER SYRUP

- 2 cups water(480 mL)

- ½ cup brown sugar(100 g)

- 2 tablespoons fresh ginger, peeled and sliced

DOUGH

- 1 ¼ cups glutinous rice flour(155 g), ¼ cup boiling water (60 ml) ¼ cup room temperature water (60 ml)

- pink food coloring

Preparation

1. Make the fillings: Add the sesame seeds to a small nonstick pan. Cook over low heat, stirring often, until they start to smell nutty, 3–4 minutes.

2. Transfer the sesame seeds to a small food processor with 2 tablespoons of sugar. Process until the seeds break down into a thick, cohesive paste. Add 1 tablespoon of butter and process until smooth. Transfer to an airtight container and refrigerate until hardened, at least 1 hour or up to 4 days.

3. Clean the bowl of the food processor, then repeat the toasting and blending process with the peanuts, remaining 2 tablespoons of sugar, and remaining tablespoon of butter. Transfer to an airtight container and

refrigerate until hardened, at least 1 hour or up to 4 days.

4. Divide the sesame paste into 10 equal portions, about 1½ teaspoons each. Repeat with the peanut paste. Freeze until ready to use.

5. Make the brown sugar ginger syrup: Add the water, brown sugar, and ginger to a small saucepan. Cook over medium-low heat, stirring occasionally, until the sugar is dissolved, 3–5 minutes. Remove the pan from the heat and let cool to room temperature, then refrigerate until ready to serve. (Alternatively, if you prefer to serve the tang yuan in hot syrup, cover to keep warm until ready to serve.)

6. Make the dough: Add the glutinous rice flour to a large bowl. Slowly pour in the

boiling water and whisk until combined. Slowly pour in the room temperature water and stir with a rubber spatula until the dough comes together. Turn the dough out onto a clean surface and knead with your hands until smooth and soft, 2–3 minutes.

7. Divide the dough in 2 portions. Set one portion aside and cover with a damp paper towel, then return the other portion to the bowl used to make the dough. Add a couple of drops of pink food coloring and knead with your hands (wear latex gloves to avoid dyeing your hands pink) until the color is evenly distributed.

8. Roll each color of dough into 10 equal balls, about 1 tablespoon each. Place on a tray and cover with a damp paper towel to keep from drying out as you roll.

9. Working one at a time, flatten each dough ball into a 2-inch circle. Press your thumb into the center to make a divot, then add one of the chilled filling balls to the divot and pull the dough around to encase. Roll a few times to create a smooth, uniform round. Repeat with the remaining dough and fillings, covering the filled tang yuan with a damp paper towel as you finish.

10. Bring a large pot of water to a boil. If serving cold, prepare an ice bath in a medium bowl and set nearby. Add about 6 tang yuan and immediately stir to prevent sticking. Cook until they start to float, about 3 minutes, then cook for 1 minute more. Use a slotted spoon to remove from the water and transfer to the ice bath, if applicable. Transfer to a serving bowl. Repeat with the remaining tang yuan.

11. Pour the chilled brown sugar ginger syrup over the tang yuan and serve immediately.

12. Enjoy!

Citrus Poppy Muffins With Candied Kumquats

Ingredients

for 12 servings

CANDIED KUMQUATS

- 1 cup granulated sugar(200 g)

- 1 cup water(240 mL)

- 5 kumquats, thinly sliced crosswise, seeds removed

CITRUS POPPY MUFFINS

- nonstick cooking spray, for greasing

- 5 kumquats

- 4 tangerines

- 5 large meyer lemon

- 1 ¼ sticks unsalted butter, room temperature, plus 2 tablespoons

- 1 cup granulated sugar(200 g), divided, plus 5 tablespoons

- ½ teaspoon kosher salt

- 2 large eggs

- 2 large egg yolks

- 1 ¾ cups all purpose flour(215 g)

- 2 tablespoons buttermilk

- 1 ½ tablespoons poppy seeds

- 1 tablespoon vanilla extract

- 1 ½ teaspoons baking powder

Preparation

1. Make the candied kumquats: Prepare an ice bath in a medium bowl and set to the side with a medium fine-mesh strainer.

2. Bring a small pot of water to a boil, then add the kumquats and blanch for 1 minute. Immediately pour through the fine-mesh strainer, then set the strainer with the kumquats in the ice bath to shock (this will help keep the bright orange color of the kumquats).

3. In the same small pot, combine the sugar and water and cook over medium heat until the sugar dissolves, 2–3 minutes. Add the kumquats and reduce the heat to low. Simmer for 20–30 minutes, until the kumquats are soft and translucent. Use a small strainer or fork to remove the kumquats from the syrup and transfer to a wire rack to dry, making sure that none of the slices are touching. Let cool completely. Set the pot aside.

4. Make the citrus poppy muffins: Preheat the oven to 375°F (190°C). Generously grease a standard or mini muffin tin with nonstick spray.

5. Zest the kumquats, tangerines, and Meyer lemons into a small bowl. Set the citrus aside.

6. In the bowl of a stand mixer fitted with the paddle attachment, cream together the butter, 1 cup sugar, the salt, and citrus zest on medium-high speed until light and fluffy, about 2 minutes. Scrape down the sides of the bowl.

7. Reduce the mixer speed to low speed and add the eggs and egg yolks, 1 at a time, mixing to incorporate between each addition.

8. Turn the mixer off and add the flour, buttermilk, poppy seeds, vanilla, and baking powder. Mix on low speed until just barely combined; do not overmix.

9. Use an ice cream scoop to scoop batter into the prepared muffin tin, filling each cavity half to three quarters of the way full.

10. Bake the muffins until the edges are golden brown and a toothpick inserted into the center comes out clean, 12–15 minutes for regular muffins or 8–11 minutes for mini muffins.

11. Meanwhile, add the remaining 5 tablespoons of sugar, the zested kumquats and tangerines, and juice of the zested Meyer lemons to a blender. Blend on low speed until the mixture is a chunky purée.

12. Pour the purée into the same pot used to candy the kumquats. Bring to a simmer over low heat and cook for about 5 minutes, until the sugar is dissolved. Remove from the heat and let steep until ready to use.

13. Once the muffins are done, remove from the oven. Set a wire rack over a baking sheet and place this upside down on top of

the muffins. Carefully flip the upside down to turn the muffins out of the pan while still hot, then quickly flip them right-side-up on the rack. Strain the citrus purée to remove the solids, then use a pastry brush to brush a thick layer of the purée on top of each muffin while they are still warm. Before the glaze dries, decorate the tops of the muffins with the candied kumquats.

14. The muffins are best the day they are made, but any leftovers will keep tightly wrapped at room temperature for up to 2 days.

15. Enjoy!

Sata Andagi

Ingredients

for 50 servings

- oil, for frying

- 6 cups all purpose flour(750 g)

- 3 cups sugar(600 g)

- 2 tablespoons baking soda

- ½ teaspoon salt

- 6 large eggs

- 1 cup whole milk(240 mL)

- ¼ cup orange(60 mL)

- 1 pinch of orange zest

Preparation

1. Fill a deep pot or skillet with enough oil to come 2 inches (5 cm) from the top of the pan. Heat the oil over medium heat until it reaches 350°F (180°C).

2. In a large bowl, whisk together the flour, sugar, baking soda, and salt.

3. Stir in the eggs, milk, and orange juice. Mix until a thick batter forms.

4. Add the orange zest and mix to incorporate.

5. Using a cookie scoop or tablespoon, drop ping pong ball-size dough balls into the hot oil.

6. Fry for about 5-7 minutes, or until golden brown. The doughnuts should float to the surface when they are done.

7. Drain on a paper towel-lined plate.

8. Serve hot.

9. Enjoy!

Sweet Potato-Pecan Cinnamon Rolls

Ingredients

for 12 servings

ROLLS

• 1 cup plain unsweetened soy milk(240 mL), or other non-dairy milk

- ¼ cup vegan butter(55 g)

- 1 cup mashed sweet potato(250 g), from 1 baked medium sweet potato

- 3 cups unbleached all-purpose flour(375 g), plus more for dusting

- ¼ cup granulated sugar(50 g)

- ½ teaspoon salt

- 2 ¼ teaspoons active dry yeast, 1 packet

- ½ teaspoon grapeseed oil

FILLING

- ½ cup brown sugar(110 g), or coconut sugar, or a mix of the two

- ½ tablespoon ground cinnamon

- ¾ cup toasted pecans(95 g)

- ⅓ cup vegan butter(75 g)

SWEET POTATO CREAM CHEESE FROSTING

- ½ cup vegan cream cheese(110 g)

- ½ cup confectioners sugar(80 g)

- ¼ cup mashed sweet potato(60 g), from ¼ baked medium sweet potato

- ½ teaspoon pure vanilla extract

Preparation

1. In a small saucepan, warm the soy milk and vegan butter over medium heat until the butter has melted. Do not boil it. Remove from the heat and stir in the mashed sweet potato.

2. In a large bowl, mix together the flour, granulated sugar, salt, and yeast. Pour the liquid **ingredients** into the dry and use a wooden spoon to combine. Once it gets too difficult to stir, use your hands to combine the ingredients.

3. Flour a clean work surface and transfer the dough onto the prepared work space. Knead it until you've got a smooth dough ball. Lightly oil a large bowl. Place the dough ball in it, cover with plastic wrap or a kitchen towel, and let rise for 1 hour. The dough should double in size.

4. Make the filling: In a small bowl, combine the brown sugar and cinnamon and set aside. Chop the pecans into small pieces and set aside. In a small saucepan, melt the vegan butter and set aside.

5. Once the dough has doubled in size, preheat the oven to 375°F (190°C).

6. Press the air out of the dough, then transfer it back onto your floured work space. Roll the dough until it is about ¼-inch (6 mm) thick. You should end up with a roughly rectangular oval, about 12x16 inches (30x40 cm).

7. Brush the dough with the melted butter, sprinkle with the cinnamon-sugar mix, and then top with the chopped pecans. Fold the short side of the dough over and roll tightly until you have a log.

8. Carefully cut the log into twelve 1-inch (2 cm) slices. Grease a large skillet or a 10-inch (25 cm) round baking dish and place the rolls in it cut-side down.

9. Bake for 25 minutes, or until they've expanded and turned slightly golden on top.

10. Meanwhile, make the frosting: Place all the **ingredients** in a food processor or standing mixer with the whisk attachment on high and blend until creamy.

11. Remove the rolls from the oven and let cool for 5 to 10 minutes. Top with the sweet potato frosting and serve immediately. They will stay fresh for up to 2 days, but they're best eaten the day you bake them.

12. Enjoy!

Healthier Key Lime Bars

Ingredients

for 16 servings

CRUST

- ¾ cup almond flour(70 g)

- 3 tablespoons coconut oil

- 3 tablespoons honey

- ½ teaspoon ground cinnamon

- 1 pinch salt

FILLING

- 14 oz cans of coconut milk, chilled overnight

- ½ cup lime juice(120 mL), from about 2 limes

- ⅓ cup honey(110 g)

- 2 limes, zested

Preparation

1. Line an 8-inch (20 cm) square baking dish with parchment paper to hang over the edges.

2. Make the crust: in a medium bowl, combine the almond flour, coconut oil, honey, cinnamon, and salt. Mix with a spatula until smooth.

3. Transfer the crust to the baking dish. Use a spatula to smooth the crust into a thin, even layer covering the bottom of the pan. Set aside.

4. Make the filling: open the cans of coconut milk and use a spoon to scoop the thick cream at the top of the can into a medium bowl. Set aside the remaining liquid for another use, such as in smoothies, soups, or sauces.

5. Beat the coconut cream with a hand mixer until very fluffy, about 5 minutes.

6. Add the lime juice and honey. Continue to beat until smooth and fluffy, about 2 minutes.

7. Pour the filling over the crust and use a spatula to smooth out the top.

8. Top with the lime zest.

9. Freeze for at least 2 hours, until the filling has set.

10. Grab the parchment on both sides and lift the frozen bar from the baking dish. You may need to use a knife to release the edges or turn the dish upside down on a cutting board and tap on the bottom to release the block.

11. Quickly cut the block into 16 2-inch (5-cm) square bars.

12. Enjoy!

Dairy-Free Pumpkin Spice Panna Cotta

Ingredients

for 4 servings

- ¾ cup raw cashews(95 g)

- warm water, for soaking

- coconut oil, for greasing

- 1 ¼ cups water(300 mL)

- 1 pinch of kosher salt

- 6 tablespoons maple syrup

- ⅓ cup unsweetened pumpkin puree(75 g)

- 1 tablespoon pumpkin spice

- ¼ cup hot water(60 mL)

- 1 teaspoon agar agar

- ground cinnamon, for garnish

- cinnamon stick, for garnish

Preparation

1. Add the cashews to a medium bowl. Pour in enough warm water to completely cover the cashews, then soak for at least 2 hours, or overnight. Drain.

2. Grease 4 4-ounce ramekins with coconut oil and set aside.

3. Add the cashews to a blender with the water and a pinch of salt. Blend on high speed for 2 minutes, or until very creamy.

4. In a medium saucepan over medium-low heat, combine the cashew cream, maple syrup, pumpkin puree, and pumpkin spice. Warm slowly, stirring occasionally, until the sugar is dissolved and the mixture is simmering.

5. Add the agar agar to hot water and stir until there are no lumps and the agar agar is fully dissolved.

6. Pour the agar mixture into the warm cashew cream and whisk to combine. Increase the heat to medium, bring to a gentle boil, and whisk continuously for 3 minutes, until thickened. Remove from the heat and immediately divide between the greased ramekins. Smooth the tops.

7. Refrigerate for at least 30 minutes. (The agar will set at room temperature, but chilling the panna cotta in the fridge will expedite the process.)

8. When ready to serve, use an offset spatula or butter knife to carefully work around the edges of the ramekins to loosen the panna cotta. Invert onto serving plates

and garnish with ground cinnamon and cinnamon sticks.

9. Enjoy!

Hidden Heart Strawberry Bundt Cake

Ingredients

for 8 servings

CAKE

• 2 loaves vanilla pound cake

• 16 tablespoons unsalted butter, room temperature

• 1 ½ cups sugar(300 g)

• ½ teaspoon kosher salt

- 1 teaspoon vanilla extract

- 3 large eggs

- 3 cups all-purpose flour(375 g)

- 2 teaspoons baking soda

- ½ cup whole milk(120 mL)

- ½ cup strawberry puree(165 g)

- nonstick cooking spray

VANILLA SIMPLE SYRUP

- ¼ cup water(60 mL)

- ¼ cup sugar(50 g)

- ½ tablespoon vanilla extract

WHITE CHOCOLATE GANACHE

- 1 cup white chocolate chip(175 g)

- ½ cup heavy cream(120 mL), hot

FOR DECORATING

- red sprinkle

- pink heart sprinkle

SPECIAL EQUIPMENT

- heart shaped cookie cutter

Preparation

1. Preheat the oven to 350°F (180°C).

2. On a cutting board, slice the ends off the pound cakes, then slice the cakes to the same thickness as the heart-shaped cookie cutter.

3. Cut the centers out of the slices of pound cake with the cookie cutter. Set the hearts aside and discard the scraps or save for another use.

4. In a large bowl, cream the butter, sugar, and salt with an electric hand mixer for 4 minutes, or until fluffy. Scrape down the sides of the bowl with a rubber spatula.

5. Add the vanilla and eggs, 1 at a time, beating to incorporate before adding the next. Scrape down the sides of the bowl again.

6. Sift in the flour and baking soda, then fold to incorporate a bit with a rubber spatula.

7. Continue mixing with the electric hand mixer, streaming in the milk and beating

until just incorporated. Add the strawberry puree and beat to combine.

8. Grease a bundt pan with nonstick spray.

9. Add 2 cups of cake batter to the bundt pan and smooth the top with a spatula. Place the pound cake heart cut-outs around the pan, points up, submerging in the batter by about ½ inch (1 ¼ cm.) Add the rest of the batter, then gently tap the pan against the counter 2-3 times to release any air bubbles.

10. Bake for 45 minutes, or until a toothpick inserted in the center of the cake comes out clean. Let the cake cool for 30 minutes, then invert onto a wire rack set over a baking sheet.

11. Make the vanilla simple syrup: In a small saucepan over medium heat, combine the

water, sugar, and vanilla. Cook until the sugar is completely dissolved and the mixture reaches a gentle boil. Remove from the heat and set aside to cool.

12. Make the white chocolate ganache: In a medium bowl, pour the heavy cream over the white chocolate chips. Whisk until completely smooth.

13. Using a skewer, poke holes all over the cake, then brush with the vanilla simple syrup.

14. Pour the white chocolate ganache over the cake. Decorate with sprinkles.

15. Slice the cake to reveal the hidden hearts, then serve.

16. Enjoy!

Grilled Peach And Blueberry Cobbler

Ingredients

for 8 servings

FILLING

- ¾ cup granulated sugar(150 g)

- ⅓ cup all purpose flour(40 g)

- ½ teaspoon kosher salt

- 1 lemon, juiced

- 1 lemon zest

- 1 vanilla bean, split lengthwise and seeds scraped

- 4 cups blueberry(400 g)

- 4 cups peaches(900 g), sliced

BISCUITS

- 2 cups all-purpose flour (250 g), plus more for dusting

- ¼ cup granulated sugar (50 g)

- 2 tablespoons baking powder

- 1 teaspoon kosher salt

- 1 stick unsalted butter, frozen

- 1 cup buttermilk (240 mL), plus 1 tablespoon, cold, divided

- 1 tablespoon turbinado sugar

- Vanilla ice cream, or whipped cream, for serving

Preparation

1. Make the filling: In a large bowl, whisk together the sugar, flour, salt, lemon juice and zest, and the vanilla bean seeds.

2. Add the blueberries and peaches and use a spatula to toss until well coated.

3. Transfer the filling to a 10-inch (25 cm) cast-iron skillet. Refrigerate until ready to top.

4. Make the biscuits: In a large bowl, whisk together the flour, granulated sugar, baking powder, and salt.

5. Using a cheese grater, grate the cold butter into the flour mixture. Working quickly, use your hands to toss the butter in the flour.

6. Pour 1 cup (245 ml) of buttermilk into the flour mixture and use a spatula to stir into a shaggy dough.

7. Turn the dough out onto a lightly floured surface. If the dough looks too wet, dust with a bit more flour. Form the dough into a 5x7-inch (12 x 17 cm) rectangle, and sprinkle with more flour. Fold the dough in half, then roll out again. Repeat 4–5 more times to build the flaky layers of the biscuits.

8. Add a few tablespoons of flour to a small bowl. Dip a 2-inch (5 cm) round cookie cutter in the flour, then punch out 16 biscuits, pressing the cutter straight down. Reroll the dough as needed to cut out more biscuits.

9. Arrange the biscuits on top of the fruit filling, making sure they are touching. Brush

the biscuits with the remaining tablespoon of buttermilk and sprinkle with the turbinado sugar. Refrigerate until ready to grill.

10. Preheat the grill to 350°F (180°C).

11. Place the cast-iron skillet on the grill and shut the lid. Grill the cobbler for 1 hour 15 minutes, until the biscuits are golden brown and the filling is bubbling.

12. Let sit for 30 minutes at room temperature, then serve with ice cream or whipped cream.

13. Enjoy!

Double-Sided Cookies

Ingredients

for 40 cookies

OATMEAL CHOCOLATE CHIP COOKIES

- 1 ½ cups all purpose flour(185 g)

- 1 ½ teaspoons baking soda

- 1 teaspoon kosher salt

- 1 cup old fashion oat(100 g)

- 1 ½ sticks unsalted butter, softened

- 1 cup light brown sugar(220 g)

- 1 teaspoon vanilla extract

- 1 large egg

- 1 cup chocolate chips(175 g)

CHOCOLATE PEANUT BUTTER COOKIES

- 1 ½ cups all purpose flour(185 g)

- ¼ cup cocoa powder(30 g)

- 1 ½ teaspoons baking soda

- 1 teaspoon kosher salt

- 1 stick unsalted butter

- 1 cup creamy peanut butter(240 g)

- 1 cup light brown sugar(220 g)

- 1 teaspoon vanilla extract

- 1 large egg

Preparation

1. Preheat the oven to 350°F (180°C). Line 2 baking sheets, or as many as you have, with parchment paper.

2. Make the oatmeal chocolate chip cookie dough: In a medium bowl, sift together the flour, baking soda, and salt. Add the oats and stir to incorporate, then set aside.

3. In a large bowl, cream together the butter, brown sugar, and vanilla with an electric hand mixer on medium speed until smooth, about 3 minutes. Add the egg and beat to incorporate.

4. Add the dry **ingredients** to the wet **ingredients** and mix until just combined. Add the chocolate chips and fold to

incorporate with a rubber spatula. Set the dough aside.

5. Make the chocolate peanut butter cookie dough: In a medium bowl, sift together the flour, cocoa powder, baking soda, and salt. Set aside.

6. In a large bowl, cream together the butter, peanut butter, brown sugar, and vanilla with an electric hand mixer on medium speed until smooth, about 3 minutes. Add the egg and beat to incorporate.

7. Add the dry **ingredients** to the wet **ingredients** and mix until just combined.

8. Scoop 1 tablespoon of oatmeal cookie dough and 1 tablespoon of peanut butter

cookie dough and roll together in a ball. Repeat with the remaining dough.

9. Place the cookies at least 2 inches (5 cm) apart on a baking sheet, press down lightly to flatten, and bake for 12 minutes, or until golden brown. Let cool for 10 minutes.

10. Enjoy!

Honey-Glazed German Apple Cake

Ingredients

for 12 servings

• 1 ½ sticks unsalted butter, softened, plus more for greasing

- 1 ½ cups all purpose flour(185 g), plus more for dusting

- 1 cup sugar(200 g)

- 1 ½ teaspoons lemon zest

- 2 large eggs

- 1 ½ teaspoons vanilla extract

- 1 ½ teaspoons kosher salt

- 1 ½ teaspoons baking powder

- 2 sweet tart apples, such as honeycrips

- 1 tablespoon honey

- 1 ½ teaspoons water

Preparation

1. Preheat the oven to 335°F (170°C). Grease a 9-inch (22 cm) tart pan (with a removable base) with butter, then dust with flour, turning to coat evenly and tapping out the excess.

2. In a large bowl, cream the sugar, butter, and lemon zest together with an electric hand mixer until light and fluffy, 2–3 minutes.

3. Make a well in the center of the creamed sugar and butter. Add the eggs, vanilla, and salt to the well. Beat to combine.

4. Sift in the flour and baking powder, then beat just to incorporate. The batter will be thick and sticky.

5. Using a rubber spatula, transfer the batter to the prepared tart pan and spread in an even layer, starting at the center and working toward the outer edges.

6. Cut lobes off of the apples, then discard the cores.

7. Stick a skewer crosswise through the flat side of each apple wedge, just deep enough so the skewer is not exposed; this will prevent the knife from cutting all the way through the apple. Set the apples flat-side down and thinly slice lengthwise, stopping your knife when you hit the skewer. Remove the skewers.

8. Arrange the apples in a circle pattern over the batter and gently push in to submerge slightly.

9. Bake the cake for about 45 minutes, or until a toothpick inserted in the center comes out almost completely clean. The cake will brown around the edges before it's done.

10. In a small bowl, mix together the honey and water.

11. Brush the honey mixture over the top of the warm cake.

12. The cake can be served immediately, but it is even better the next day, as the apples will infuse the cake with their flavor when left to sit covered at room temperature overnight. Remove the tart ring, then slice and serve.

13. Enjoy!

Peanut Butter Keto Cookies

Ingredients

for 14 cookies

- 2 cups almond flour(250 g)

- 6 tablespoons keto friendly powdered sugar substitute

- 1 large egg

- ½ teaspoon kosher salt

- 1 cup natural salted crunchy peanut butter(240 g)

- ½ cup unsalted butter(115 g), melted

Preparation

1. Preheat the oven to 350ºF (180ºC) and line 2 baking sheets with parchment paper.

2. In a large bowl, mix together the almond flour, powdered sugar substitute, egg, salt, peanut butter, and melted butter until thoroughly combined.

3. Scoop the dough into 14 balls using a ¼ cup ice cream scoop and place on the prepared baking sheets. Flatten the cookies by crossing 2 forks on top and pressing down slightly.

4. Bake the cookies for 10–12 minutes, turning the baking sheet halfway, until fragrant and slightly golden. Remove the cookies from the oven and transfer to a wire rack to cool.

5. The cookies will keep in an airtight container at room temperature for up to 4 days.

6. Enjoy!

CHAPTER 6: INCORPORATING LIFESTYLE CHANGES

Cushing's disease can be controlled and the patient's quality of life improved by dietary and lifestyle adjustments. Alterations to one's way of life can alleviate symptoms, boost the efficacy of medications, and encourage better health overall.

Including regular physical activity as part of your new lifestyle is crucial. Individuals with Cushing's disease might benefit greatly by engaging in moderate-intensity aerobic activities such as brisk walking, swimming, or cycling. It has positive effects on cardiovascular health, muscle strength, weight management, and mental and emotional well-being. Exercise plans should be tailored to each person's strengths and limitations with the help of their healthcare providers.

The ability to control stress is also important. Individuals with Cushing's disease may already have elevated cortisol levels, but stress can make these levels much higher. As a result, learning and employing stress-reduction strategies is crucial. Relaxing activities can be anything from meditation and deep breathing to yoga and other hobbies. Finding beneficial stress-reduction strategies may have a profound effect on health.

Managing Cushing's illness also requires sufficient sleep. Develop a relaxing nighttime ritual and stick to a regular sleep schedule. Sleep well to aid the body's recuperative processes and enhance your health.

In addition, it is crucial to keep your family and friends close. Having people who care about you and are willing to help you through the tough times is essential when you have Cushing's disease.

Last but not least, it's important to do your part in managing your disease by keeping yourself informed. Maintain constant contact with your healthcare team, go to all scheduled visits, and strictly adhere to your treatment plan. That way, if your symptoms or treatment options ever alter, you can react quickly.

The management of Cushing's disease and the promotion of general health and well-being can benefit from incorporating these lifestyle changes in addition to dietary alterations. Never hesitate to seek the counsel of medical experts for advice tailored to your specific condition and needs.

Printed in Great Britain
by Amazon